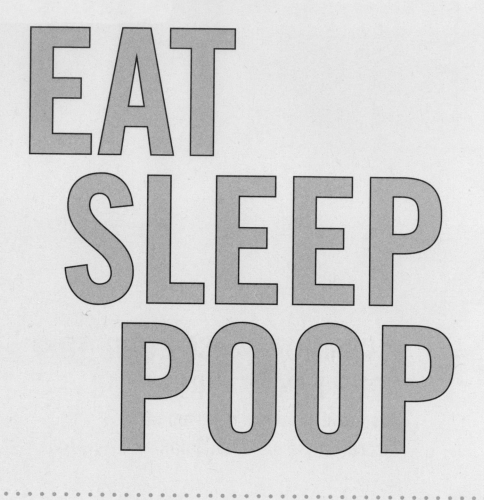

A COMMON SENSE GUIDE TO YOUR BABY'S FIRST YEAR—

Essential Information from an Award-Winning Pediatrician and New Dad

SCOTT W. COHEN, M.D., F.A.A.P.

SCRIBNER

New York   London   Toronto   Sydney

Scribner
A Division of Simon & Schuster, Inc.
1230 Avenue of the Americas
New York, NY 10020

For my daughter, Aubrey Grace

CONTENTS

INTRODUCTION

· ·

L ike most new parents, you will probably be inundated with parenting advice during the first year of your baby's life. When she
sneezes or spits up or has a fever, you'll not only receive unso-
licited guidance from friends and family, you'll also be tempted to
click on to countless informational websites where it can be overwhelming to sort through the sage and not-so-sage advice. And
as happens after most Internet searches, you'll likely end up with
more questions than answers. That's why I've written this book: to
answer your questions about caring for your baby and to be your
commonsense pediatrician-in-residence.

What do I mean by common sense? The philosophy behind *Eat,
Sleep, Poop* is what I call *Common Sense Parenting*. It basically boils
down to this: raising a child should be enjoyable and as stress-free
as possible. The most current science and medicine are certainly
important when dealing with your baby's health and well-being,
but so is parenting in a way that feels comfortable and makes sense
for your family. I want you to be able to use common sense in raising your baby so that health and safety fit in easily with the fun of
having a child. And trust me: *it is fun,* as well as challenging.

Although humankind has been raising children for a very long
time, in this age of overstressing and overparenting, some parents
and doctors would have you believe that caring for a child requires
systematic calculations, precise schedules, and the input of a host

of experts. I believe that informed common sense is your best tool. During this fascinating first year of your baby's life, I want to empower you to look at your child's green poop and smile rather than worry; to calmly treat a temperature of 102 knowing that everything will be okay; and to have faith that your baby will learn to sleep through the night without holding a grudge against you.

Eat, Sleep, Poop will give you answers to such new-parent questions as: What should I feed her when she's ready to eat solids? How often should she take a nap? Why does she have a fever? Why is she crying for no reason? What's that crusty rash on her scalp? And it will also help you figure out when you can handle something on your own and when you should contact your doctor. Included in the back of the book is a section of fact sheets that you can photocopy or tear out for easy reference to help you quickly answer your most common concerns.

I know from personal experience what it's like to be a first-time parent, because my wife and I recently welcomed our first daughter, Aubrey, into the world. This book was written during Aubrey's first year of life and our first year as parents. I now scrutinize my own advice as a doctor and find myself questioning some of it as a dad. That's why you'll find my "Daddy vs. Doctor" confessions throughout the book, which hopefully will convince you that doctors are human, too. Even when we know the right thing to do, sometimes our hearts and emotions tell us otherwise. After all, it's one thing to advise your patients to let a baby learn to self-soothe by crying through the night. It's another to be the dad listening to his little girl cry for three nights straight.

I developed the ideas behind my Common Sense Parenting philosophy by reflecting on how my parents raised my siblings and me. They didn't have medical degrees, but somehow my mom and dad survived our rashes, whooping cough, vomiting, and diarrhea. Looking back, I sometimes wonder how I'm even still here. I tumbled down the stairs in a plastic egg-shaped walker I called my "Vroom Vroom." I slept on my stomach. I played in the snow without gloves or a hat. I ate Play-Doh and dirt and dog food. I slept in the same bed as my brother and sister until I was eight. But somehow my parents navigated through it all by applying a little common sense and we turned out just fine. I think their brand of common sense involved knowing when to worry and when not to. When they were worried, they called the doctor. Otherwise, they felt confident they knew what to do.

It is my hope that *Eat, Sleep, Poop* will give you that kind of confidence so you can enjoy the adventure you're about to begin.

Scott Cohen, M.D., F.A.A.P.

CHAPTER 1

PREPARE

Save the Date

• •

The period before your first baby is born is one of the most excit-ing times in your life, but also one of the most anxiety-producing and nerve-racking. As anxious parents-to-be, we try to control a situation that is already out of our control, and we find it nearly impossible to focus on what is most important—looking forward to the baby's arrival. In this chapter I'm going to help you focus by offering Common Sense Parenting advice on preparing for your baby's arrival. Hopefully, you'll then be able to cut down the anxiety and concentrate on the excitement.

Here's what we'll focus on:

- What to buy
- How to choose a pediatrician
- Cord blood banking
- What to bring to the hospital

Nesting—What to Buy

If you're like most couples, as soon as you find out you're hav-ing a baby, you are immediately inundated with advice. Everyone with kids tells you what you absolutely must buy for the first year. Unfortunately, most first-time parents have trouble cutting anything from the list of "must have" baby items, which is why many end up with a bedroom like my friends'.

I remember visiting them shortly after the birth of their first child. They took me on a tour of their new apartment, and when we walked into their bedroom, the three of us could barely squeeze in among all the baby paraphernalia. Along with their queen-sized bed, the room was cluttered with a crib, a co-sleeper, a sleep nest, and a bassinet, all of which they said they bought because everyone told them they absolutely had to have them. My friends worried that if they didn't buy everything everyone had recommended, they wouldn't be properly prepared and their child might suffer. As it turned out, their baby ended up sleeping in their bed with them for the first six months, leaving all of the baby contraptions unused. Now they look back and laugh. Like many other well-meaning first-time parents, my friends had allowed their anxiety to overwhelm them.

I have to admit: I was also one of those anxiety-ridden first-time dads who fell into the too-much-stuff trap. When my wife and I were preparing for the arrival of our child, it seemed like we were constantly buying new stuff for the baby. In every store we went to, the salesperson would tell us what we needed to buy and then point to a wall of infant items that appeared to reach to the sky. Even though many of the suggested articles seemed to perform the exact same function, we bought them anyway. Our baby's room soon became the most expensive room in the house.

So how can you prevent the too-much-stuff scenario? The following is a list of Newborn Must-Haves. The purpose of this list is not to tell you what kind of crib or bottle to buy, but to make sure that you remember to buy one. These items are the Common Sense Parenting essentials; anything you choose to add to the list is up to you. In the resources section at the end of the book you'll find a handy checklist that you can tear out or photocopy.

Newborn Must-Haves Checklist

Sleep

___ Crib

___ Crib mattress

___ Mattress pad cover
___ Fitted sheet

Crib: You are soon going to realize that all your baby does is eat, sleep, and poop. And of the three, the one you'll yearn for the most is sleep. It goes without saying that your child needs a place to sleep, but there's no need to give her more than one place to do that. Decide where you would like your infant to sleep, and go with your decision. You may decide that you want to put her crib in your room because it will be easier for you to get to her in the middle of the night when she needs to be fed. You may want her right next to you in a co-sleeper (a small, portable crib that sits next to your bed). Or you may choose to have her sleep in her own room in her own crib from the start. I do feel that routine and repetition are very important, so the sooner you start the routine, the better. Ultimately, if the goal is to have her sleep in her crib and in her own room, the transition will be easiest on both you and her if you start in that location.

Common Sense Bottom Line
Select an item for your baby to sleep in and go with it; she will not need three different places to sleep. The earlier she is in her own bed the better.

Mattress: I remember visiting a popular baby store when we were getting ready for our daughter. We were in the mattress aisle overwhelmed by the thirty mattresses leaning up against the wall ranging in price from eighty to eight hundred dollars. We called over a salesperson and asked, "Which mattress do you recommend?" He responded, "We tell our customers to ask their pediatrician." My wife whimsically smacked me on the arm and we started to laugh. The salesperson asked, "What's so funny?" and I said, "I'm a pediatrician, but I don't remember a course in medical school entitled 'Sealy versus Serta.'"

We ended up basing our decision on common sense (no need to go overboard and buy the most expensive mattress) as

7

well as my pediatric training (a firm mattress reduces the risk of SIDS).

Common Sense Bottom Line

Choose a crib mattress that is firm, as it will reduce the risk of SIDS. As for organic versus nonorganic . . . I'll leave that up to you.

Travel

___ Car seat
___ Stroller
___ Diaper bag

Car seats: Imagine four grown adults hovering around a plastic car seat staring blankly like a bunch of cavemen confronting a television for the first time. I used to say that you had to be a rocket scientist to figure out how to install a car seat until one of my patients, who worked for NASA, threw in the towel. And just like asking for directions, any father would rather spend eight hours trying to install this simple device than ask for help.

When we went to buy our first car seat, the car we drove to the store wasn't the car we'd be installing the car seat in. So the staff couldn't help us with the installation. No problem, I thought. I'll just watch as the store manager gives me a quick demonstration and then I'll do it when I get home. After the half-hour demo, I was well-schooled in all the possible ins and outs, dos and don'ts of proper car seat installation. I felt like a pro. I got home, unpacked the box, and went to work. An hour later, after unproductively fiddling around with the thing, I was drenched in sweat. I pulled out the directions and tried to follow them. No luck. I called in the expert: my wife. She reread the instructions and relayed directions to me to no avail. I called the store, and after trying out a couple of their helpful tips, I got in the car, drove back to the store, and had the store manager install the car seat for me. Note to self: when you buy a car seat, drive to the store in the car into which you'll install the car seat.

Common Sense Bottom Line

Unless one or both of you is an engineer or car mechanic, go to a car seat installation center at your local police station, fire department, car dealership, or baby supply store and have a pro do it. Then drive home with a smile on your face knowing your child will be sitting safely in a properly installed car seat.

Diaper bag: In the diaper bag make sure to have diapers, wipes, diaper cream, plastic bags for dirty diapers, a changing pad, and a change of clothes. I also recommend that you keep a little bin full of the same supplies on every floor or in every major room of your house so that you can quickly tend to a dirty diaper.

Clothing
___ Onesies/sleepers
___ Swaddling blanket

Clothing: You are going to buy and receive lots of "cute" outfits for your newborn. These are more for you than for your baby. My daughter had a bigger wardrobe before she was born than I've ever had in my life. She had so many dresses with layers of lace I remember asking my wife how many balls she was planning to attend in the first year of her life. Remember, you are going to be hungry and sleep deprived, and all you'll want to do is change that diaper and go back to sleep. Going through layers of clothing will not help your stress level, so keep it simple.

Common Sense Bottom Line

I recommend investing in lots of onesies. My daughter wore them almost exclusively for the first four months. These all-in-one garments are inexpensive, easy to wash, save time for you, are comfortable for your baby . . . and cute!

Changing

___ Changing table with a pad/soft rug or mat
___ Diapers
___ Gauze/baby wipes
___ Diaper cream

Diapers: You are going to go through so many diapers that you may start having dreams about them. Disposable diapers are inexpensive and simple to use. I recommend buying them in bulk. Some infants go through ten to twelve diapers per day. If you want to go green, you can choose cloth diapers. Keep in mind, however, that while you won't be filling up a landfill with disposable diapers, the overall effect on the environment may be no different if you take into account how much water is involved in washing reusable diapers. The new cloth diapers come with waterproof diaper covers that clip or Velcro close for quick, easy use.

Diaper wipes: While some hospitals recommend using small square gauze pads and water as diaper wipes, I think this is a challenging test for new parents. Try and scrape off tarry newborn poop with a tiny gauze pad! I have seen parents use a whole stack for one diaper change. Yes, your child's skin is sensitive; and yes, we do want to decrease the risk of an allergic reaction. But *baby wipes* are safe and very effective. Choose a wipe that doesn't have a lot of extra additives or fragrances, as this will decrease the risk of irritating your newborn's skin.

Diaper creams: These are used to treat or prevent diaper rash, which every baby will get at some point—even if you are the parent of the year and change every diaper immediately. Diaper creams create a barrier to protect the irritated skin from being re-irritated by the baby's poop and pee, thus allowing the skin to heal. The thicker the cream the better. I recommend using it when you notice a rash rather than as a preventative measure. Why put it on if it's not necessary?

Note: Doctors no longer recommend using talc powders because they can be dangerous for babies to inhale.

10

Bath/Hygiene

___ Infant bathing basin
___ Sponge/washcloth
___ Baby soap and moisturizer
___ Nail file/clippers

Bathing basin: It is very difficult to hold a newborn in a sitting position while you bathe her, especially when she doesn't yet have good head and neck control. I recommend a bathing basin in which your child can lie down. This type of basin has a sling that goes over it like a tight hammock, so the baby lies in the sling and the water seeps through into the basin. This is helpful because your child is not sitting directly in the water, which reduces the risk of drowning.

Baby lotions: Just like baby wipes, baby lotions, shampoos, and soaps are safe. Parents have been using them for decades. You do not have to use them if you do not want to, but they smell good and are safe. Deciding whether to use organic or nonorganic products is a matter of personal preference. In the end, my wife and I used what our parents used on us as babies—good ol' Johnson and Johnson.

Nail files: It seems every newborn has nails like Freddy Krueger, and you'll be surprised at how often they scratch themselves. (Fortunately, a child's facial scratches will heal without scarring, so no need to worry.) Nail files tend to work better than clippers because you don't have to worry about clipping your child's cuticle, which can be painful and bleed. If you do nick her by accident, just place a little Neosporin on the cut and it should heal fine. Some nails even peel off. I recommend nail care while your child is sleeping. A moving target is always more difficult.

Medications

___ Infant and children's acetaminophen (Tylenol)
___ Children's diphenhydramine (Benadryl)
___ Electrolyte replacement fluid (Pedialyte)

11

___ Antigas/colic remedies (Mylicon, Gripe water, Hyland's
Colic Tabs)
___ Sunscreen
___ Insect repellant

Medications: I recommend stocking up on essential medications. This will save you a trip in the middle of the night when your
child is sick and needs them. I have included a dosing sheet (see
page 266) for your convenience, but you should consult with your
doctor before using any medication. Some of these medications
have a shelf life of up to one year, but check their expiration date
prior to using.

- *Infant Tylenol Concentrated Drops* (generic: acetaminophen) will be helpful if your child has a fever or is in
  pain.
- *Children's Benadryl* (generic: diphenhydramine) is helpful
  for allergic reactions.
- *An electrolyte replacement fluid* such as Pedialyte can be used
  to rehydrate after a vomiting or diarrheal illness.
- *Colic and gas remedies* are not medically proven but are safe
  and may be helpful. Half of my patients say they are great,
  while the other half find them useless. *Mylicon drops* are
  like Gas-X for babies. *Gripe water* and *Hyland's Colic Tabs*
  are homeopathic mixtures that may be soothing to your
  child's stomach. *Chamomile tea* is also a good remedy to
  try. These remedies can be found at most supermarkets or
  drugstores and come with a dropper. You can give these to
  your child several times a day. Follow the package directions for dosing frequency.

Sunscreen lotion: This can be used before six months of age, but
it is best to keep your infant out of direct sunlight for the first
couple of months. If you do go out in the sun, use a sunscreen with
an SPF of at least 30 (most children's sunscreen lotions have at
least SPF 50), and apply early and often.

> **Common Sense Bottom Line**
> *Stock your medicine chest with medications for common baby ailments so you'll have them available before you need them.*

Accessories
___ Digital thermometer (rectal and axillary/underarm)
___ Pacifier
___ Bulb syringe
___ Saline nasal spray
___ Gum/tooth cleansers
___ Hand sanitizer

Thermometers: Do not buy an expensive, fancy thermometer. (If you get one as a gift, return it for a nice credit at the store.) Ear and temporal artery thermometers are expensive but inaccurate. Invest in an inexpensive digital rectal thermometer. These thermometers are accurate and easy to use, and display results in eight to twenty seconds. The accuracy of the thermometer is very important. This is because the difference between 100.3 and 100.4 degrees Fahrenheit in a child under two months of age may be the difference between seeing your doctor in the office or going immediately to the hospital for a battery of unpleasant tests. With infants under two months old, always use a rectal thermometer, as they are the most accurate. Once your child is over two months of age, you can use an axillary (underarm) thermometer. Oral thermometers can be used when your child is five years old.

Pacifiers: I am often asked whether or not to give a baby a pacifier, and, if so, what type. In general, I feel if you can find a way to soothe your child without one, a pacifier is one less thing you'll have to wean them off of in the future. On the other hand, if a pacifier soothes your child, and it gets you a couple of extra hours of sleep or quiet time, then it is probably worthwhile. Although I would not introduce one for this purpose alone, pacifier use while sleeping may decrease the risk of SIDS because it keeps the baby

13

in a more aroused state. So, if she is already using a pacifier, think of it as an added bonus, and don't worry: Just because your infant uses a pacifier doesn't mean she'll still need it when she's three. As for choosing a pacifier: don't waste your money on fancy ones. Your baby won't care if she's sucking on a freebie from the hospital or a hundred-dollar Swarovski crystal model. And when it comes to the touted orthodontic pacifiers, keep in mind that pacifier use does not affect permanent dentition or negatively affect the palate unless used after the age of three.

Common Sense Bottom Line
If you can find a way to soothe your baby without a pacifier, you'll have one less thing to wean her off. If you do introduce one, inexpensive is just as good as fancy.

Bulb syringe: In general, newborns sound congested. On top of that, they are going to get a lot of colds in the first few years of life. Since there is no medication that has been proven to successfully relieve cold symptoms in children under the age of four, you may turn to saline drops and bulb suction. However, even if your child sounds like Darth Vader, try to resist the urge to use the suction too often.

Common Sense Bottom Line
If you see something in your infant's nose and that something is bothering her, suck it out with a bulb syringe. Otherwise leave it alone. Every time you stick the syringe in her nose, it will irritate the inside lining, causing more swelling and congestion. If it is not bothering her, don't let it bother you.

Hand sanitizer: If you are going to be Type A about anything, then be neurotic about hand washing. Fever and illness will stop both you and your baby in your tracks, so it's not a bad idea to carry hand sanitizer in case there isn't a sink available to wash your hands. Keep anyone overtly sick or coughing and sneezing away from your baby. School-age children, especially toddlers, who are sticking their hands in their mouth or nose, are always brewing something. They don't need to be kissing your newborn.

Feeding
___ Bottles (4 ounces)
___ Nipples (level one)
___ Breast pump
___ Freezer bags
___ Nursing pads
___ Nursing bra

Bottles and Nipples: Most infants take 2 to 4 ounces every 2 to 4 hours for the first 2 to 4 months of their life. Do not invest in a lot of larger bottles initially; you won't need them. And there's no need to go crazy buying a bunch of different bottle nipples. If milk comes out of the nipple and your child gets it, that's all that matters. Start with a level-one nipple because it mimics the flow of breast milk the best. As your child gets older or if you notice she is getting frustrated with the slow flow, then increase to a faster-flow nipple. My daughter was still happily using a level-one nipple at one year of age. As for sterilization: you may want to sterilize or boil bottles and nipples in hot water prior to the first time you use them, but after that you can safely hand wash them with soap and water or throw them in the dishwasher. You do not have to sterilize bottles or boil them in hot water after each use. After all, do you know of a breast that is sterile? Be realistic . . . but if you want to sterilize, be my guest.

Breast pumps: Breast pumps range in price from a couple hundred dollars for the electric kind to less expensive hand pumps. Hospital-grade electric pumps, which are the fastest, may cost as much as four hundred dollars to rent for five months. Consider your time. In the middle of the night when you want to go back to sleep you probably want a fast pump. Although hospital-grade may not be necessary, a hand pump may be tediously slow.

What's Up Doc?—How to Choose a Pediatrician

Once you know your due date, it's not too early to start shopping around for a pediatrician. Choosing the right one can be a daunting task. Whoever you select will be the person overseeing the health of your pride and joy for the first twenty-one years of her life. Here are some tips to help you pick the right person for the job.

Where to Start

If you are new to your area, call your local hospital and speak to the nurse in charge of the pediatric ward or the newborn nursery, and ask which pediatricians she recommends. The charge nurse sees these doctors every day and knows how they interact with their patients and the hospital staff. They know who is cranky before their first cup of coffee and who is always smiling. You could also visit a local chat room for new moms. I have found that parents will gladly spread the news, both good and bad, on doctors in the area.

If you know the area, ask friends, family, or your own doctors—especially your obstetrician—for a recommendation. This is one time when lots of outside advice is welcome. Consider the personalities and expectations of the people giving you suggested names. The more you have in common with these folks, the more likely the pediatrician they recommend will be a good match.

Once you have a list of prospective pediatricians, visit their offices and meet with them. Many pediatricians do prenatal interviews. This is a chance for you to get to know the doctor and his philosophies, as well as take a look at the office. Some doctors will meet with you privately, one on one, while others do a more informal group session with several sets of parents. I am a fan of group sessions because they allow you to hear the concerns of other parents as well as questions you may not have thought to ask.

Just as you would never buy a car without doing your homework and test driving it first, you should not only speak to potential doctors but also be knowledgeable about their practices. Remember, this will be a long relationship and you want it to be as comfortable a fit as possible. So consider the following factors.

Office Size

Inquire as to how far in advance the doctor is booked. This will give you an idea of how hard it may be to get an appointment. The number of doctors in an office, as well as the number of exam rooms, will help you figure out how long you might be stuck in a busy waiting area. There should be at least two exam rooms per doctor.

How large is the waiting area? This is where you are going to spend most of your time with your anxious child and other noisy little ones. A waiting room that is large and fun may offset the wait time, compared to a small crowded waiting area. A smaller office, on the other hand, may have a more personal feel.

Age

A young doctor may be more up-to-date on current procedures and treatment options than an older doctor, but will not have the same amount of practical experience. The key is not how old the doctor is, but his willingness to ask for help when it is needed and refer to a specialist if required. You might consider a younger doctor if you want your child to have the same physician throughout childhood, since an older doctor may retire before your child is grown.

Gender

Some parents think a girl should have a female doctor and a boy a male doctor. Although this may be true for older children and teenagers who have a hand in picking a new doctor, your pediatrician's gender should not matter if your child has been with that doctor since birth. Your child will grow up with her doctor and her trust in that person will grow as well. What's most important is that you choose someone with whom you feel comfortable.

Common Sense Bottom Line
Don't worry about choosing a male doctor for your baby boy or a female doctor for your baby girl; go with the person you feel most comfortable with. Patient-doctor trust will deepen with time.

Board Certification

You should make sure that your pediatrician is board certified. You can easily find out by asking the doctor or looking on his business card for the initials F.A.A.P., which stands for Fellow of the American Academy of Pediatrics. You can also go to the American Board of Pediatrics website at www.abp.org. Board certification means that your doctor has kept up to date with the field and taken a test to prove it. Pediatricians need to recertify every ten years by written examination.

Availability

Most doctors have standard nine-to-five hours Monday through Friday, but it is important to know whether your prospective pediatrician has office hours on weekends or in the evening, which may save you a trip to the emergency room or urgent care. Most doctors will make themselves available by phone, and many are accessible via e-mail. Ask your physician if he is available by phone or e-mail and how quickly he is able to respond. Also inquire as to the availability of nurses or other support staff for phone consultation.

If there are multiple doctors in a practice, ask if your child will always see her primary physician, or if she will often be seen by others in the practice. Some practices share patients and you see whoever is available, while in other practices you almost always see one doctor. I believe that seeing one primary doctor ensures continuity of care. However, you may need to see other doctors in an emergency or when your child is sick.

Who Is On Call After Hours?

Many practices alternate being on call (answering patient questions after hours) with the other doctors in the office, while some practices share this responsibility with other groups. As a result, you may not know the person to whom you are speaking, and he may not practice medicine in the exact same manner as your doctor. Some offices utilize nursing triage companies that follow a standard protocol book. This tends to be less personal, and studies have shown that more families are sent to the emergency department as a result.

Overall Philosophy

Vaccines, antibiotics, and alternative therapies such as homeopathic or holistic medicine are all issues that may be important to you, so try to find a doctor with a similar philosophy. Some physicians require vaccines be given at the recommended age, while others may allow you to spread them out. Some may offer homeopathic remedies prior to starting antibiotics. Having a similar philosophy about these issues will make office visits more productive. However, it is a good idea that both you and your doctor are open to discussing options and concerns that may veer from a particular medical philosophy.

Personality

This may be the most important factor to consider when choosing a pediatrician. Not only do you want your child's doctor to be well-trained and medically knowledgeable, but since your son or daughter will be spending the next eighteen to twenty-one years visiting this person, you'll want to make sure that those visits will be pleasant, relaxed, and educational. Some parents choose pediatricians who can just tell them what is wrong and how to fix it; it doesn't matter to them if their doctor has a personality. But you want to feel that you can talk openly with your child's physician about the health issues that concern you. You should feel comfortable speaking with your pediatrician, and hopefully, when your child is older, she will feel comfortable confiding in that person as well.

Ancillary Services

Some offices have an in-office lab that can save trips to a local hospital or lab for blood work. If your pediatrician does not have a lab, she may have nurses who are trained to draw blood, which can then be sent off to the lab without you having to make a separate trip. Another service that can be very helpful is an informational website containing handouts on pertinent topics. Your doctor's website can assure you that you're getting

19

information you can trust rather than trying to weed through a Google search.

Staff

If the office staff is not friendly and helpful, it can undercut any positive feelings you have for your pediatrician. Receptionists answer the phone when you want to make an appointment for your sick child. The billing staff are the folks you'll speak with if you cannot make a payment or are confused about a specific charge. And the nurses will be giving your child her shots and answering medical questions on the phone. The more comfortable your child feels with the nurses on staff, the more relaxed she will feel during her office visit.

Facilities

While your infant will not be as aware of the office environment as an older child, as she grows she will appreciate the kid friendliness of the pediatrician's office. Many children refer to their doctor's office as the "shot place," but the more comfortable and fun the office is, the less anxious your child will feel.

You may want to ask if there are separate entrances and waiting areas for sick and well visits, so that your healthy newborn isn't sitting next to a toddler who is coughing and sneezing.

How close and easy it is to park is also an important consideration when transporting your infant back and forth to the doctors.

Financial Responsibility

It is incumbent upon you, the patient, to discuss your financial responsibility with a potential doctor's office. Find out what insurances the doctor accepts and if he is in your insurance's network. If your pediatrician does not take your insurance, you are considered out of network and you may have to pay in full at the time of each visit.

Your newborn is on either Mom's or Dad's insurance policy for only thirty days after delivery. Make sure you call your insurance company to place your child permanently on your plan or their own plan within those thirty days. This will ensure that your child is covered without the need for underwriting. And also make sure to verify her benefits so you are not surprised when the bill comes.

Hospital Affiliation

It is important that your doctor has admitting privileges at the hospital at which you are delivering because he can see his patients there and write orders on how to treat them. He will be able to see your baby every day and is responsible for writing orders and discharging your newborn. If your child has to be hospitalized later in life, your pediatrician can take care of her in the hospital with which he is affiliated. If your pediatrician does not have privileges at the hospital where you are delivering, ask the hospital or your obstetrician whom he recommends to see your child in the interim.

Punctuality

As a child, I always dreaded waiting in the cold exam room for a half hour, naked except for that strange paper gown that never seemed to fit. You may think that a doctor who sees his patients on time is unheard of, but it's not inappropriate to ask about a pediatrician's punctuality. Doctors expect you to show up on time, so it is okay to expect the same from them (with a little leeway for emergencies).

How to Use the Following Checklist

Now that you know what to look for in a pediatric practice, use the following checklist when you speak to a prospective doctor on the phone or at a prenatal visit. Before you speak with him, sit down at home and rate the following categories from 1 (not important) to 5 (very important). Make a copy of your rated form for each pediatrician you are planning to visit. Write the doctor's name on the top of the page and take it with you to your meeting. As you learn about the office, place a check mark on the line to the left of the rating scale if the office fits that particular criterion.

When you get home, look at your check marks and see if they correspond to characteristics that you feel are most important. If so, you have found your match. If not, keep searching.

21

. . . .

Pediatrician Checklist

Name of Doctor/Office: _____

	Not important				Very Important
Office size					
___Small (three or fewer doctors)	1	2	3	4	5
___Large (more than three doctors)	1	2	3	4	5
Gender					
___Male	1	2	3	4	5
___Female	1	2	3	4	5
Age					
___Young	1	2	3	4	5
___Old	1	2	3	4	5
Board certification	1	2	3	4	5
Availability/office hours					
___Weekend hours	1	2	3	4	5
___Nighttime hours	1	2	3	4	5
Access to doctor					
___Via phone	1	2	3	4	5
___Via e-mail	1	2	3	4	5
___Office visits only	1	2	3	4	5
Who sees you in the office?					
___Your doctor	1	2	3	4	5
___Another doctor in the practice	1	2	3	4	5
___Physician assistant	1	2	3	4	5
___Nurse	1	2	3	4	5
Who takes after-hours calls?					
___Your practice	1	2	3	4	5
___Shares with another pediatric group	1	2	3	4	5

___Nursing triage or hospital	1	2	3	4	5
___No one	1	2	3	4	5
Overall philosophy					
___Western medicine	1	2	3	4	5
___Homeopathic/holistic	1	2	3	4	5
Personality	1	2	3	4	5
Ancillary services					
___In-house lab	1	2	3	4	5
___Informative website	1	2	3	4	5
___Access to specialists	1	2	3	4	5
Staff					
___Not friendly (1)/most friendly (5)	1	2	3	4	5
___Physician assistants	1	2	3	4	5
___Registered nurses (RN)	1	2	3	4	5
___Licensed vocational nurses (LVN)	1	2	3	4	5
___Medical assistants	1	2	3	4	5
Facilities	1	2	3	4	5
Financial responsibility					
___Takes your insurance (in network)	1	2	3	4	5
___Fee for service (out of network)	1	2	3	4	5
___Bills for you	1	2	3	4	5
Hospital Affiliation					
___Visits your newborn in the hospital after birth	1	2	3	4	5
Punctuality	1	2	3	4	5

Daddy vs. Doctor—Choosing a Pediatrician

During my wife's pregnancy, friends and relatives told her, "You're so lucky to have a pediatrician at home! You don't have to go through the search for a good one." But I knew that it's not the standard procedure for a physician to treat his own child, that it would be too difficult to separate my emotional attachment from what might be medically best for her. Still, I had to admit that it was going to be hard for me to relinquish control to another doctor, especially when it came to my own child. I planned to have my medical kit by the bedside so I could exam our daughter immediately after delivery.

When we started the process of selecting a pediatrician, we had the following requirements: My wife wanted someone who was warm and receptive. As a first-time parent, she didn't want to feel uncomfortable asking "stupid questions." Even though I'm a pediatrician, I wanted someone who could give my wife and me a perspective different from my own, which tends toward the more relaxed end of the scale. That way we could both rest reassured that Aubrey was getting the very best attention.

Equally as important to us was the doctor's medical training. We were thrilled to find someone who had trained at a children's hospital. In the unfortunate event of having a baby who was seriously ill, we wanted someone who had extensive experience in managing all types of scenarios.

We also wanted someone who had enough time to sit and talk with us and not make us feel that we were being rushed through appointments. And we decided that we wanted someone who was young enough so that Aubrey could have the same doctor throughout her childhood.

We chose a young, female pediatrician whose warm personality and medical expertise was just what the doctor and his wife ordered.

> After Aubrey was born, the stethoscope that I had packed in my duffel bag and brought along to the delivery room was never unpacked. I had no urge to examine her, nor did I think of her as my patient. I trusted the qualified person we had chosen as our daughter's doctor. As for me, I needed—and wanted—to focus on what was most important: being Aubrey's daddy.

What's in the Fridge?—Umbilical Cord Blood Banking

Another decision you'll be confronted with prior to delivery is whether or not to bank your child's umbilical cord blood. You are going to be inundated with mailings and brochures from companies that will offer to store the cord for a "nominal" fee. One father even asked me if he could just keep his baby's umbilical cord in his own refrigerator at home. Obviously, this is not recommended, but we should discuss the reasons why you may want to bank your child's umbilical cord blood.

The idea behind cord blood banking is to keep your newborn's healthy stem cells in case they're needed later for transplantation—that is, to replace bad cells, such as cancer cells. Although this idea may seem cut and dry, there is more to the story. Cord blood bank brochures list hundreds of illnesses for which this procedure can be curative, and yet there is the slimmest of chances that you will be able to use the banked stem cells for your child. Let me explain why.

When a child develops a malignancy such as leukemia, or a rare metabolic or autoimmune disorder, doctors usually look to irradiate the bad cells and replace them with healthy new stem cells. These stem cells can be from bone marrow or cord blood. These stem cells are often acquired from an *allogenec* donor—that is, from another individual. It is important that the donor's stem cells are as close a match to the recipient's as possible to minimize the potentially fatal risk of the recipient rejecting the donor's cells. Since a perfect match is your best bet for a successful transplant, it makes sense to use your own stem cells. Sounds simple, right? It's not. In fact, if your child came down with an illness such as leukemia, and you had saved her cord blood, the stem cells from that cord blood likely would not be used, because, most often, the condition already existed in the infant's cord blood. So the doctor would need to look for an outside donor for the stem cell transplant.

There is the possibility that with new technological advances there will be more applications for the use of cord blood. For example, using it to generate new organs or tissues. Extensive research is currently looking into the benefits of cord blood used in this way.

At the moment, however, cord blood banking is a double-edged sword. If you bank your child's cord blood and never use it, you have wasted money but possibly gained peace of mind. If you do not bank your child's blood and could have used it, you might regret it. So how should you decide what to do?

My wife is someone who loves insurance policies. We joke that if a salesperson came to our door and offered us insurance in case of the one-in-a-million chance of being struck by lightning, she would buy it. Still, when we were pregnant we were offered cord blood banking for a much-discounted rate and chose not to do so. My wife and I reasoned that, unlike most insurance, we were not likely to be able to use it in the future. We also felt that the cord blood banking companies were preying on our fears at a vulnerable time.

So, while the chances are that your child will not be able to use her own cord blood in the future, there are a few situations in which you might consider utilizing a cord blood bank:

1. If you have a family member with a known genetic or malignant medical condition that could potentially benefit from cord blood transplantation.
2. If you are someone who is going to stay up at night worrying about the slim possibility of your child being affected by an illness that may benefit from transplanting her own stem cells—and money is not an issue.

If you fit into either of these categories and choose to use a private cord blood bank, make sure the company has an institutional review-board-approved protocol with signed informed consent, and that it complies with national accreditation standards developed by the Foundation for Accreditation of Cellular Therapy (FACT), the U.S. Food and Drug Administration (FDA), and the Federal Trade Commission (FTC), as well as similar state agencies.

You should also know that there are two types of cord blood banks: *private* and *public*. Private banks are private companies that you pay to bank your child's cord blood for the sole use by your child or someone you designate it to. These banks charge a collection fee as well as a monthly or yearly holding fee. Public banks, on the other hand, bank cord blood for anyone's use, free of charge. This is similar to a blood bank. A donation to a public cord bank is a gift of life to someone who can really use it.

Common Sense Bottom Line
Cord blood banking companies are asking you to buy insurance that you will likely not need. The chances of your child needing her own cord blood stem cells range from one in one thousand to one in two hundred thousand.* And there is no evidence of the safety of such stem cell transplantations. My recommendation is that you decline the offer to store your child's cord blood in a private bank unless you fall into one of the two categories listed above. If you want your baby's stem cells to potentially help someone else, store them in a public bank.

It's Time!—The Hospital and What to Bring

Now that you've used your Common Sense Parenting smarts to get ready for the big day, think about the hospital where your newborn will arrive. Does your pediatrician have privileges at the hospital you've chosen? Does your hospital have a neonatal intensive care

---

*AAP Policy Statement, "Cord Blood Banking for Potential Future Transplantation," *Pediatrics* 119, no. 1 (January 2007): 165–70.

unit and pediatricians on staff who are available in case of emergency? These are some of the questions my wife and I had before our daughter was born. We didn't want to be in a situation where we had to be transported to another hospital for a specialist, rather than having everything at our disposal under one roof. Luckily, both our obstetrician and pediatrician had privileges at a hospital that fit these requirements, which alleviated a lot of our anxiety.

Whatever questions you might have at this point, the more you have answered prior to delivery the more empowered and less anxious you will feel. So make a list of questions that are still of concern to you, and find out the answers.

As you look forward to B-day, here are my suggestions for making sure you're ready:

- *Take an infant CPR class.* You should be able to find one at your local hospital. When you know what to do in case of an emergency, you'll feel more confident and empowered.
- *Take a tour of the hospital.* Be familiar with the labor and delivery rooms and where you are supposed to check in. Visit the newborn nursery, the rooms where you are going to stay, and where your baby is going to be taken for testing after delivery.
- *Do a mock run.* Drive from your home to the hospital along the route you plan on taking and know alternate routes in case of traffic or an emergency. Walk the exact route you plan on taking from the parking lot to the admission station. If possible, fill out a preadmit form so that you do not have to fill out paperwork when you are admitted. This is the last thing you want to be doing when you are in labor.
- *Pack your bags* and place them in the car ahead of time. Think of your hospital stay as a mini vacation. If you have trouble sleeping in another bed without your favorite pillow or blanket, bring it. You are going to be at the hospital up to two days for a vaginal delivery and up to four days for a cesarean section. Pack accordingly. To your surprise, you may even have several hours of downtime during labor. If you enjoy listening to music on your iPod, browsing the

Internet on your laptop, or reading a magazine, then pack them. Don't forget your toiletry bag, several changes of clothes and pajamas, as well as comfortable shoes or slippers. Bring an outfit and blanket that you want to put your child in for the ride home. Ask what the hospital supplies; many hospitals have diapers, onesies, swaddling blankets, hats, shampoo, soap, digital thermometers, bulb suction, and a plastic bathing basin that they will give to you to keep. Don't forget your camera and video camera. Charge the batteries and bring extra ones. This moment only happens once, and you don't want to miss it.

- *Make sure your car seat is properly installed.* You won't be allowed to leave the hospital without it.
- And finally . . . relax. Enjoy the anticipation! You're about to have a baby!

CHAPTER 2

WELCOME

Before Your Baby Comes Home

• •

You've waited nine long months for this day to arrive. Your bags are in the trunk of your car, the baby's car seat is properly installed in the backseat, and you're good to go. As you pull out of the driveway, you take one last glance at your home knowing that it will never look the same.

You arrive at the hospital, where they begin to monitor your contractions and tell you that today's the day. A wave of cool sweat envelopes you and a combination of emotions swell. You are anxious, scared, and elated all at the same time.

Your doctor tells you to start pushing and you begin to see the head appear. You are overwhelmed with tears of joy and driven to push harder. And then, as if the hours of hard labor could be so easily erased, there is a peaceful calm as you are handed your new baby.

Welcoming your child to the world is a joyful yet overwhelming experience. To ensure that you're not overly overwhelmed by what routinely takes place in the hospital following her birth, in this chapter I'll familiarize you with the following procedures:

- Apgar score
- Antibiotic eye ointment
- Umbilical cord care
- Vitamin K shot
- Baby's first bath

- Hearing screen
- Newborn screen
- Circumcision

And I'll also address the special circumstances surrounding premature births.

What If My Baby's Not a Perfect Ten?—The Apgar Score

As parents, we're too often obsessed with rankings: the top ten preschools, the All-Star Little League lineup, the highest SAT scores. It seems everyone wants his or her child to score the highest and run the fastest. Parents' concern for their newborn's Apgar score, an assessment of an infant's health immediately after birth, is no different. I have had parents anxiously ask me why their child didn't get a perfect ten on the Apgar score, as if they were competing in the Olympics. As you may have guessed, however, an Apgar score does not predict your child's future college—or preschool—acceptance. So what is an Apgar score?

The Apgar score allows physicians to quickly assess a newborn's physical condition after delivery and to determine any immediate need for extra medical or emergency care. The assessment is based on five categories scored from 0 to 2 with the highest total score being a ten. The five categories are:

	0	1	2
Color	blue	blue extremities (acrocyanosis)	pink
Muscle tone	floppy	some flexion	active movement
Heart rate	none	less than 100	more than 100
Respiratory rate	none	weak cry	strong cry
Psychomotor agitation (response to agitation)	no response	grimace	strong cry, withdrawal

The score is calculated mentally by the nurse or doctor taking care of the infant in the labor and delivery room at one, five, **31** and ten minutes of life, then documented in the newborn's chart. Several factors may affect the score: medications the mother has been given and ongoing interventions that are being made on the infant. For example, many infants are initially floppy or have blue arms and legs at birth during their transition to the outside world, which will lower their initial Apgar score. However, after the doctor warms the baby with blankets and vigorously stimulates her by rubbing, these issues usually resolve and the subsequent Apgar score is much higher. If the mother had been receiving a medication, such as magnesium to slow contractions or lower high blood pressure, the infant may initially have depressed respirations or poor muscle tone until the medication wears off. This should not be a reason for the mother not to take this medication if it is needed. Even if your baby's initial Apgar score is low, with supportive measures, or merely time, the score will improve. The important thing to remember is that it is the final score that matters. If the initial score is five and the final one is nine, the nine is what's important. Remember, too, that it is very difficult to score a perfect ten. The "judges" are always taking off a point for color, tone, or cry.

Common Sense Bottom Line
Can your infant have a less-than-perfect Apgar score and still be perfect? Yes.

Daddy vs. Doctor—A Perfect Score

After my daughter was born, the nurse turned to me (knowing I was a pediatrician) and asked me what I had calculated Aubrey's Apgar score as. I had not even thought about it. It didn't matter. She came out, she started to cry, and everything else was a blur. I looked at her lying in my wife's arms: sure her arms and legs looked blue and her face and nose were smooshed, but she was perfect. As a father I gave her a ten. As a pediatrician she scored a nine. Numbers? Not really where it's at.

Do I Have to Put That Slimy Stuff in My Baby's Eyes?—Antibiotic Eye Ointment

Shortly after birth, most infants receive antibiotic eye ointment to prevent eye infections from gonorrhea and chlamydia, which are a major cause of blindness in newborns. These bacteria may infect the newborn during passage through the birth canal, and although it is less common, they can also be acquired during cesarean section. Silver nitrate drops were commonly used until the early 1980s when erythromycin or tetracycline ointment became the standard of care. These antibiotics have few side effects and rarely cause irritation to the eyes. Parents frequently ask me, "I know that we don't have gonorrhea or chlamydia, so can we just skip the eye ointment?"

If you know that you and your spouse do not have these two sexually transmitted diseases, then you are probably fine going without the medication. However, there is very little risk associated with the application of the antibiotic and a large upside: it will also prevent other bacterial eye infections.

Common Sense Bottom Line
I am a big believer in prevention, so I recommend the use of antibiotic eye ointment. Remember: big upside, small downside.

Why Are They Painting Her Umbilical Cord That Strange Color?—Cord Care

Many parents remember the brilliant blue-green triple dye that is often painted on an infant's umbilical cord in the hospital. Why the colorful attention to this no-longer-needed part of a newborn's body? Shortly after your child's birth, the obstetrician will clamp and cut the umbilical cord, leaving a small umbilical stump, which eventually dries up and falls off. As the stump dries up, it is the perfect entryway for bacteria to enter the body and cause infection. Studies have shown that bacteria may be carried from infant to infant by hospital caregivers in the nursery. Since such an infec-

33

tion can be severe, a number of topical agents have been used, with varying degrees of success, to decrease infection and speed up separation of the umbilical stump. The list includes: breast milk, 70 percent alcohol, salicylic sugar powder, micronized green clay powder, colloid silver-benzyl-peroxide powder, neomycin-bacitracin powder, 1 percent basic fuchsine, and the colorful triple dye.

So far, no study has found a decrease in infection rate with the use of any antibiotic ointment, compared with simply cleaning the cord with soap and water—otherwise known as *dry cord care*. On the other hand, several studies have demonstrated that application of certain topical solutions does have an affect on separation time. Separation of the umbilical stump ranges from about five days with breast milk, seven days with powders, eight days with nothing, ten days with alcohol, twelve days with antibiotics, and anywhere between one to two weeks with triple dye. The variation in timing of cord separation is not significant enough to recommend one treatment over another. However, the American Academy of Pediatrics (AAP) and the World Health Organization (WHO) recommend dry cord care as the preferred method of umbilical cord care. Again, spot cleaning the cord with soap and water to remove any debris or poop will sufficiently minimize the risk of infection.

What else can you do to decrease the risk of infection to your infant's umbilical stump? Consider having your baby "room in" with you to lessen the possibility of her being contaminated by bacteria in the nursery. This will also allow for skin-to-skin contact between mother and baby, which promotes colonization of normal healthy bacteria from the mother's skin.

Common Sense Bottom Line
Topical solutions do not decrease the risk of infection to your newborn's umbilical stump. They may, however, delay cord separation. If your hospital offers a topical cord treatment and your infant is going to spend time in the nursery, then I recommend it. Otherwise, simply spot clean. But do notify your doctor immediately if there are any signs of redness or swelling around the umbilical stump.

Why Does She Need This Shot Now?—The Vitamin K Shot

Parents hate the idea of giving their child shots, especially immediately after birth. But most agree that if a shot will prevent spontaneous bleeding it is a worthy reason to poke their child. Of all the routine procedures that are offered to your infant, this is the most important. This injection is so important, in fact, that most hospitals make families sign a waiver if they refuse it.

Vitamin K helps blood to clot. All infants are born deficient in vitamin K, and breastfed infants remain deficient longer because breast milk is a poor source of vitamin K. Without a vitamin K injection, there is an increased risk of an infant spontaneously bleeding anywhere in her body, even the brain. Vitamin K deficient bleeding (VKDB) may occur early (within the first week of life) or late (between two and twelve weeks of age). Is it common? No. But why take a chance? The vitamin K shot—a simple intervention—can eliminate the risk altogether.

Some parents worry about possible side effects of the shot and wonder about alternatives, such as administering vitamin K orally to the infant or having Mom take a vitamin K supplement hoping it will be transmitted to the baby. Unfortunately, these alternative therapies are not effective. First of all, the absorption rate of oral vitamin K differs from person to person, which means we can't actually determine the amount entering the body. Although oral vitamin K has been shown to decrease the incidence of early bleeding, it does not decrease the incidence of late bleeding. Second, maternal supplementation with vitamin K does not improve clotting times in infants, nor does it decrease the rate of intraventricular bleeding (bleeding into the brain).

Common Sense Bottom Line

The vitamin K injection is a must! Other than the immediate pain of the injection and some possible redness around the injection site, the risks of the vitamin K injection are minimal.

Does She Really Need That Natural Moisturizer?
—Baby's First Bath

In most hospitals, after you have had a chance to bond with your infant, a nurse will ask if it is okay to take your baby for her first bath. This may seem like a simple question, but many parents choose to forgo the bath in order to preserve the *vernix*, a white, cheesy coating covering the infant's skin. Vernix begins to be produced at the end of the second trimester, and it acts as the skin's protective covering against prolonged amniotic fluid exposure. (Think of what happens to your skin when you spend too much time in the bath and multiply that by several months.) After birth, the vernix acts as another protective barrier between the infant and the outside world.

Comprised mainly of water, vernix is a natural emollient that not only moisturizes the skin and keeps it clean but also has antimicrobial proteins that help protect against bacterial penetration. With so many beneficial functions why would anyone want to wash it off?

There are many different approaches to bathing an infant after birth. Some people are proponents of gently removing blood, meconium, and other soil but leaving the vernix intact. Others use water and gentle soap or antibacterial cleanser to gently clean the skin and remove unwanted debris as well as the vernix. No method has been proven more beneficial than another. Despite the antimicrobial properties of the vernix, studies have not shown a decrease in infection rates when it is left intact.

In healthy full-term infants, I recommend delaying the first bath and bonding with your newborn. After you have bonded, let the nurse bathe your infant with warm water and a gentle soap to remove the blood and meconium, as well as the vernix. It's my feeling that your infant's skin provides a sufficient barrier to prevent infection and that it is safe to use a topical moisturizer. In other words, the vernix is no longer needed.

Common Sense Bottom Line

Accept the nurse's offer to give your baby her first bath—during which blood, meconium, and the vernix are gently removed.

Can She Hear Me Now?—The Newborn Hearing Screen

Some parents worry about their infant's hearing if they call her name and she doesn't look at them. Or if they clap their hands loudly and the baby doesn't turn her head toward the noise. Although these behaviors can be normal for infants who hear perfectly well, sometimes the anxiety over an infant's hearing is justified.

Out of every one thousand infants in the United States two to three are born deaf or hard of hearing. For that reason, I recommend having your child's hearing checked soon after birth. Early detection of a hearing loss with the universal hearing screen means children will have better language outcomes because of significantly earlier referral, diagnosis, and treatment.

It is easiest if the hearing screen is completed in the hospital prior to your infant's discharge, so ask your hospital ahead of time whether or not a hearing screen will be performed. Fortunately, most hospitals perform these screenings routinely. If not, ask them to refer you to an audiologist or early-hearing detection center, and have an initial hearing screen performed in the first month of your child's life.

One of two hearing tests is used to screen infants:

1. *the otoacoustic emissions test* (OAE), or
2. *the auditory brain stem response test* (ABR).

During the OAE test, the examiner plays clicks or tones through a tiny probe placed just inside the ear canal and the response or echo is measured. If no echo is found, it may indicate a hearing loss. The ABR test measures the brain's response to sound directly.

During this test your child wears headphones and the examiner places three electrodes on different parts of her head. As sound is played through the headphones, the electrodes measure electrical activity from the stimulated brain. A lack of activity may signal a hearing deficit.

Both of these exams are painless, fast, and usually performed when your child is asleep. If your child does not pass her newborn hearing screen you will be referred to a testing center where confirmatory testing can be performed by a hearing specialist or audiologist. The confirmatory testing should be completed during the first three months of life. Just because you are referred to a specialist does not mean that your child cannot hear. Repeat testing will be performed and if your child passes, no further evaluation is needed. However, if the test is failed again, the audiologist, in conjunction with a pediatric ear, nose, and throat doctor (otolaryngologist), can assess the degree of hearing loss and refer your child for appropriate interventional services.

Common Sense Bottom Line
Make sure your child's hearing is tested in the first month of her life. The earlier the diagnosis, the better.

What's a PKU?—The Newborn Screen

Before your infant is discharged from the hospital she will receive the newborn screen, sometimes referred to as the PKU. All children born in the United States receive the newborn screen. In fact, PKU, or *phenylketonuria,* is just one of several diseases that the newborn screen can test for. If any of the tests come back positive, a simple medication or dietary change will likely eliminate the problem. On the other hand, if the tests are not given and a disease is not diagnosed in a timely manner, it could be devastating.

For instance, if an infant is diagnosed with *congenital hypo-*

thyroidism and is started on a medication such as Synthroid in the first two weeks of life, she will likely lead a normal healthy life as long as she takes her medication. On the other hand, if the treatment is not started promptly, the child could suffer severe repercussions including mental retardation and developmental delays.

The newborn screen is conducted using blood from a heel prick after your child is twenty-four hours old. The number of diseases screened for depends on the state in which you live and ranges from four to more than fifty. If your state only screens for a couple of diseases, you can ask to be directed to a private company that will perform a more comprehensive expanded screen.

If one of these tests returns a positive result, do not panic. Doctors will run a more specific test for confirmation. If this test comes back positive, it will be upsetting, I know. But the sooner you are aware of any health risks, the sooner you can take steps to control them and give your child the care she needs. Forewarned is forearmed.

Common Sense Bottom Line
The newborn screen is required for good reason. Don't worry; odds are everything will be negative. If further testing is advised, take the necessary steps to address your child's health concerns as early as possible.

Is This Common Surgery Really Necessary?—Circumcision

Circumcision is one of the oldest known surgeries, and many religions, cultures, and ethnicities offer their own reasons to perform or not to perform this procedure. The current policy from the American Academy of Pediatrics (AAP) reflects forty years of research and states that the benefits of circumcision are not significant enough to recommend it as a routine procedure. The decision to circumcise your son is a personal one, but it should also be an informed one. So here are the facts:

Infection/Cancer

- Circumcision decreases the risk of certain sexually transmitted diseases, such as HIV, human papilloma virus (HPV), and syphilis. In fact, circumcision has been shown to decrease HIV transmission by up to 50 percent in areas with a high HIV rate such as Africa. Since HPV is the causative agent of cervical cancer, circumcision reduces the risk of cervical cancer in women as well.

- Circumcision decreases the risk of acquiring a urinary tract infection. Urinary tract infections are four to ten times greater in uncircumcised males in the first year of life. However, urinary tract infections are usually not life-threatening and can be treated safely with antibiotics. Furthermore, the incidence of urinary tract infections in males is low to begin with.

- Circumcision decreases the risk of penile cancer. However, penile cancer is extremely rare, and even in uncircumcised males the risk continues to be extremely small.

Hygiene

- Both circumcised and uncircumcised penises require proper hygiene. The key is to know how to take care of your son either way (see Chapter 3 for further information).

Surgical Risks and Pain

- Circumcision is a surgery with relatively low risks, the most common of which is minor bleeding. Other risks, such as infection, damage to adjacent structures such as the urethra, or partial amputation are extremely rare.

- There is a possibility that the infant may need a revision of the circumcision. Unfortunately there are bad circumcisions that need to be redone or adhesions or skin bridges that need to be broken.

- Similarly, an uncircumcised individual may need a circumcision in the future if he has recurrent infections or a *phimosis* or *paraphimosis*. A phimosis is when the foreskin of the penis will not retract, resulting in a sealed cover over the head of the penis, which prevents urine from flowing freely. A paraphimosis, on the other hand, involves foreskin that remains retracted, creating a tourniquet effect around the penis, which causes extreme pain and swelling. Both of these conditions are medical emergencies that require immediate intervention and may lead to a future circumcision. Whether you are circumcised or not, the risks are about equal for needing a future surgery. Fortunately these risks are small.

- Just like you and me, infants feel pain, so a proper anesthetic should be used during the procedure. Your infant may receive a local injection to numb the area or an application of a numbing cream. Both work adequately and most infants cry during the procedure because of the position they are forced to stay in rather than the pain of the operation. After the circumcision your pediatrician can order Tylenol to control any fussiness or discomfort. Usually infants are a little clingier after the circumcision and want to feed or sleep more frequently. Either way, they are usually fine by the next day, as if nothing happened.

Sexual Pleasure

- Some groups argue that circumcision causes a dulling in the sensation over the head of the penis and as a result decreases sexual pleasure. This is a subjective conclusion and probably the least of your concerns when assessing whether to circumcise your newborn.

Peer Pressure

- Finally, there are psychosocial considerations. In addition to religious and cultural beliefs, maybe Dad wants his son to look like him. Or perhaps you are concerned about your son being made fun of in the locker room if he looks different from than the rest of his friends. These are all important concerns to consider.

41

Common Sense Bottom Line

The choice is yours. Although the data are divided, I feel that there are some legitimate benefits to circumcision, and I would consider it for my own son. I have put together a Circumcision Cheat Sheet below to help you decide.

Circumcision Cheat Sheet

	Circumcised?	
	Yes	No
Decreases sexually transmitted disease	X	
Decreases urinary tract infections	X	
Decreases risk of penile cancer	X	
Less to take care of	X (later in life)	X (as infant)
Sexual pleasure	?	?
Psychosocial	X	X
No risk of initial surgery		X
Possibility of future surgery	X	X

Will Her Early Arrival Cause Problems?—Preemies and the NICU

Any infant born fewer than thirty-seven weeks gestation is considered premature. Most infants born at thirty-five to thirty-seven weeks gestation spend about two to four days in the newborn nursery and then go home like their full-term counterparts, but some preemies need to stay in the hospital longer for monitoring in the neonatal intensive care unit (NICU). While in the NICU, some premature infants need to be monitored closely for breathing and feeding issues as well as infections.

Although dealing with the NICU may seem frightening at first, if you know what to expect, you'll feel more relaxed and more in control of the situation. Think of the NICU stay as a roller-coaster ride. There may be some ups and downs before you reach the end:

bringing your baby home—which generally happens when she reaches thirty-seven to forty-one weeks gestation.

Here are some typical concerns and common terminology relating to preemies and a stay in the NICU.

Breathing

Some premature infants require respiratory support shortly after birth. If an infant has labored breathing, she will be evaluated for respiratory distress syndrome (RDS). RDS is caused by a paucity of surfactant, a chemical produced by the lungs to decrease surface tension in the lungs and make it easier for the lungs to expand. The goal for treating RDS is simple: help her breathe until she can do it on her own. There are three major types of breathing assistance:

- *Nasal canula:* This is the most common and least invasive form of respiratory assistance. The nasal canula consists of two small plastic prongs that are placed in the baby's nose to deliver a gentle stream of oxygenated air.
- *CPAP:* If more help is needed, CPAP, or *continuous positive airway pressure,* is used. CPAP is administered through a face mask or nasal prongs, which delivers a more forceful stream of air to assist the infant in expanding her lungs.
- *Intubation:* In the most severe cases, the infant will have a tube inserted in her mouth to the upper airway or trachea and be hooked up to a ventilator to help her breathe. Sometimes surfactant is given through this tube to help improve her lungs' elasticity.

As the infant's lungs grow stronger, she will be weaned off respiratory assistance.

It is not uncommon for premature infants to have drops in oxygen saturation (*desaturations*) or to stop breathing altogether for fifteen seconds or longer (*apnea*). These events are typically caused by an immature respiratory center. They are usually short-lived and may resolve spontaneously or require stimulation such as rubbing the infant gently or an increase in supplemental oxygen.

Sometimes desaturations or apnea may happen several times a

43

day. They seem scary, but they do not deprive the brain of oxygen long enough to cause any permanent damage—and they usually disappear as the infant approaches full term. Imagine holding your breath several times a day. It may make you light-headed, but it will not cause any long-term problems. However, some infants are given a medicinal version of caffeine, which decreases the number of episodes or resolves the problem.

Heart Rate

It is normal for the heart rate of preemies to slow for brief periods of time. This condition is called *bradycardia* and generally resolves as the infant approaches full term. It will not cause long-term problems nor does it indicate that there are heart problems.

In general, apnea, desaturations, and bradycardia in premature infants are to be expected. There are, however, several situations in which these conditions may indicate the possibility of other medical concerns. For example, if the events always occur with or after feeding, they may be a sign of *gastroesophageal reflux,* or GERD (see page 89). Or, if the events increase in frequency or severity, they may be a sign of infection or anemia and your doctor will run some tests to evaluate her.

Infection

Since premature infants are at greater risk of infection, in the NICU they often will be started on antibiotics prophylactically. In other words, they are treated for a possible infection until one can either be identified or ruled out. If an infection is identified, the antibiotics will be continued until it resolves. If no infection is identified after two or three days, the antibiotics are usually stopped. To help assess whether an infection is present, blood tests will likely be taken.

Feeding

Most infants do not gain the coordination to suck on a breast or bottle nipple until thirty-four weeks gestation, so preemies generally require alternative forms of nutrition. Most begin with intravenous nutrition until the child's stomach can tolerate food. Next, the infant will graduate to *gavage feedings,* meaning a small tube is placed in her nose or mouth through which breast milk or formula can be gently advanced into the stomach. The infant will be fed through this tube very slowly at first, gradually increasing the volume and frequency as the child tolerates it. This may take anywhere from a couple of days to several weeks. Meanwhile, the NICU will monitor the infant for any digestive difficulties. Typical problems include undigested food left in the stomach, a distended abdomen, or vomiting. It is not unusual for such problems to occur—so try not to worry!

Finally, around thirty-three to thirty-four weeks gestation, your child will begin *non-nutritive sucking:* sucking on the breast or pacifier to gain strength and coordination prior to feeding by mouth. Feeding by mouth uses a lot of an infant's energy so she will be started very slowly, advancing as she tolerates the feedings. How well an infant can feed by mouth with no lingering issues generally determines when she will be allowed to go home.

Miscellaneous NICU Concerns

Now that you have an honorary doctorate in neonatal medicine and an overview of common NICU concerns, I want to highlight two more tests that your child may be given: *head ultrasound* and *ophthalmologic exam.*

- In infants who are extremely premature, usually fewer than thirty-two weeks gestation, a screening *head ultrasound* will be ordered to rule out an *intraventricular hemorrhage* (IVH), or bleeding in the brain. Premature infants are at a greater risk of bleeding because of fragile blood vessels in the brain that may break when exposed to changes in blood flow and oxygen levels shortly after birth. A head ultrasound is a simple, noninvasive test that can be performed at the bedside. If there is no evidence of bleeding, no further workup is needed, unless the infant shows clinical signs of IVH, which include an increase in apneas and bradycardias, anemia, seizures, poor muscle tone, decreased activity, or a bulging fontanelle. If a bleed is identified, it

45

will be graded on a scale of one to four, with four being the most severe. More than 90 percent of grade-one and -two hemorrhages resolve spontaneously and do not have any long-term consequences on the brain. In grade-three and -four bleeds, however, there may be damage to the brain, which may lead to such short-term conditions as *hydro-cephalus* (cerebrospinal fluid in the ventricles of the brain) or long-term issues such as cerebral palsy and learning disabilities.

An *ophthalmologic eye exam* is a routine procedure in infants fewer than thirty-two weeks gestation or extremely low birth weight infants who weigh less than 1,500 grams. The eye exam helps to rule out *retinopathy of prematurity* (ROP), which occurs when abnormal blood vessels grow and spread throughout the retina, the tissue that lines the back of the eye. These abnormal blood vessels are fragile and can leak, scarring the retina and pulling it out of position, which may lead to visual impairment and blindness. ROP is divided into five stages with the fifth stage being the most severe. Stage one or two ROP usually resolves spontaneously without treatment. The ophthalmologist will perform serial eye exams to monitor the infant's progress. More severe cases of ROP may require laser treatment or even surgery.

Common Sense Bottom Line
If your baby is born premature and brought to the NICU, she may need to go through a number of procedures and tests that can be trying for a new parent. Know that most likely everything will be fine. And be there for her!

CHAPTER 3

EXAMINE

Checking Out Your Baby from Head to Toe

. . . .

I can't tell you the number of parents who've told me that if they hadn't seen their child being born, they would have questioned whether the baby was really theirs. Having imagined a cherubic face with big blue eyes, they were instead shocked by their infant's cone-shaped head, swollen eyes, and smashed-in nose. Many a father has taken me aside to ask "if everything was okay" with his cone-headed purple baby.

In this chapter I'll put your mind at ease by explaining why your baby's initially odd appearance is perfectly normal, and I'll walk you through the nuances of an infant's body so that you'll know what to expect when you check out your new baby from head to toe.

Your pediatrician will also be checking out your newborn. He or she will perform your child's first pediatric exam within twenty-four hours after birth. So let's take it from the top—just as your pediatrician will.

Head

Again, your baby's face and head may not have the adorable round-ness you had expected. The crammed quarters of the uterus may distort her facial features so that she resembles a would-be featherweight champ after twelve rounds. But have no fear. Everything will snap back to its normal shape over the next couple of weeks. Here are some specific things you may notice about your baby's head.

She's a Conehead

You may notice swelling on the back of her head—the result of being pushed and squeezed through a small opening. This swelling may be in the form of a large, soft bump that crosses the midline anywhere on the top or back of the head (called a *caput succedaneum*). Or you may notice a lump on one side of the head (likely a *cephalohematoma*—basically a big bruise). Neither of these will affect the brain in any way.

If your child's delivery was assisted by a vacuum, you may see a target-like swelling where the suction cup of the vacuum was stuck to the scalp. Again, nothing to worry about.

Common Sense Bottom Line

None of these swellings are serious nor will they affect brain development. They'll go away after a few days or weeks and will not leave a scar. Cephalohematomas may exaggerate jaundice, or the yellow color of the skin—so notify your doctor if your child's coloring begins to turn yellow.

He Has More Holes Than a Bowling Ball

You may feel two soft spots on the top of your child's head. These are called *fontanelles* and are located on the top back (posterior) and top front (anterior) part of the head. These allow the skull to expand with the growing brain. The posterior soft spot is usually closed at birth, so you may not feel it. If it is present, it will close on its own by three months of age. The anterior soft spot, which you can usually feel as a small, soft divot, remains open until nine to eighteen months of age. You may notice the soft spot pulsating at times because there is blood flow underneath.

Common Sense Bottom Line
The soft spots are normal and will close in good time, so don't be afraid of them. You can touch the spot gently and it will not hurt your infant.

Ruffles Have Ridges—and So Does My Baby's Head!

Your infant's head is not perfectly smooth; it has ridges. Don't be alarmed. These are suture lines where the plates that make up the skull have been pushed together and overlapped due to your child's tight intrauterine positioning. As the brain and skull expand, these ridges usually flatten out, but don't be surprised to find different lumps and bumps on your child's skull.

Common Sense Bottom Line
We all have differently shaped heads and nobody's is perfectly smooth. That's why hair was invented.

Why Does She Look Like Friar Tuck?

If your baby is born with hair, you may notice her developing a bald patch in the back from lying on one spot. Then, as she loses her newborn hair, you may see the front sides receding like male-pattern baldness and the back with a semicircular patch of hair. All infants lose their hair; however, infants born with a full head of hair usually do not go fully bald because the new hair grows in quickly.

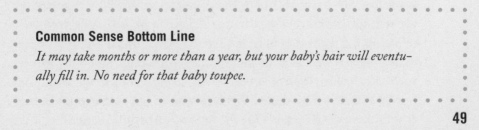

Common Sense Bottom Line
It may take months or more than a year, but your baby's hair will eventually fill in. No need for that baby toupee.

Eyes

When your infant is born she has 20/200–20/800 vision and can see best at a distance of about six to twelve inches. Amazingly, however, your child can recognize your shape from across the room, and her eyesight will quickly improve to around 20/60 by four months of age.

In the first few days following her birth, your infant may not open her eyes for long periods. Like a turtle's, her eyes may be puffy and swollen from the delivery process. On top of that, the hospital will have applied antibiotic cream to her eyes shortly after birth to help prevent infection, so it may be a few days before you can stare longingly into her beautiful blues. When you do, don't be alarmed by the following.

Popeye the Sailor Man

Don't be surprised if your baby resembles Popeye—with one eye open and the other squinting shut. As long as you have seen each eye open up all the way, simultaneously or not, everything is fine. Infants commonly open one eye more than the other or keep both eyes shut for long periods during the first couple of days after birth because of eye swelling from delivery, the application of antibiotic ointment, and general transition to the outside world.

Why Is My Baby's Red Eye a Good Thing?

Although it may ruin a perfectly good photograph, your infant's red eye is a good thing. Using an ophthalmoscope, your doctor will look in your newborn's eyes for the red reflex, which indicates that light is traveling to the back of the eye (the retina) and is bouncing back with no obstruction or interruption. The doctor sees the same red-appearing eye that you often see when you get red eye in photos. An asymmetric or absent red reflex should be evaluated by an ophthalmologist immediately. It may be a sign of something obstructing the light pathway, such as a cataract, glaucoma, or a tumor such as a retinoblastoma. Your pediatrician will also shine a light in your infant's eyes to make sure that both pupils react and that the eyes move in all directions.

Parents also wonder whether flash photography will harm an

infant's eyes. Not at all. Rest assured that your baby is ready for her close-up.

Common Sense Bottom Line
Red eye is good—and flash photography is allowed.

What's Making Her Look Cross-eyed?

You may notice that your baby looks cross-eyed from time to time, like Shaq in the fourth quarter. This is due to weak eye muscles and is normal until three to four months of age. If one eye looks in one direction all the time or you notice the crossing after four months of age, then you should have your child evaluated by an ophthalmologist.

When you move an object closer to your baby's face you may notice that both eyes move inward to look at an object. This is normal. It is also normal if your child looks right through you or stares up at a light or ceiling fan with a glazed-over expression. Your baby won't fix on an object and watch it move until six to eight weeks of age.

Common Sense Bottom Line
Staring into space is normal.

What Are Those Red Lines in Her Eyes?

If you look closely, you may see red lines in the whites of your baby's eyes. These are *subconjunctival hemorrhages* or broken blood vessels. It is very common for blood vessels in the eyes to break during the pressure of birth. These may last for a few weeks then disappear and won't cause any long-term problems with your child's eyesight.

Common Sense Bottom Line
Ignore the red lines in her eyes.

Mouth

Here are a few surprises you may notice in your newborn's mouth.

There's a Pearl in Her Mouth!

Your baby may have a white bump in the middle of the roof of her mouth. The pimplelike bump is an *inclusion cyst* called an *Epstein's pearl* and has no clinical significance. Your child doesn't feel it, it doesn't hurt or affect feeding, and it will disappear on its own.

Common Sense Bottom Line
Ignore the little white bump.

Snaggletooth

Most babies are born without teeth, but occasionally an infant is born with a natal tooth, usually a lower central incisor. This natal tooth will be replaced by a primary tooth and later by a permanent one in that location. Although a natal tooth may be somewhat painful for a breastfeeding mother (until the baby learns not to bite), no intervention is needed unless the tooth is so loose that it could fall out and cause the infant to choke. If that's the case, it should be pulled by a pediatric dentist. Otherwise, your baby can show off her one gleaming, pearly white whenever she smiles.

Common Sense Bottom Line
Have a pediatric dentist evaluate your newborn's loose tooth; otherwise, ignore it.

Why Is She "Tongue-tied"?

If you look in the mirror and lift your tongue you will notice a thin, pink band of fibrous tissue, called the *frenulum,* which attaches the base of the tongue to the inside gum of the lower teeth. If your infant is born with a short or tight one, it may be difficult for her to breastfeed because her tongue won't extend far enough back to suck properly. Instead, it will rub the nipple, which will make breastfeeding painful for Mom and inefficient for the baby. If your baby's tongue looks short and you experience pain during breastfeeding, a frenulectomy may be in order. This is a simple procedure—taking only a few seconds and causing only minimal bleeding and pain—after which breastfeeding will be much more comfortable for Mom and much easier for baby.

Common Sense Bottom Line
A simple and quick procedure can correct a tiny tongue problem that may be interfering with breastfeeding.

Heart

Although most infants are born with normal-sounding hearts, some are diagnosed with heart murmurs. A murmur is a sound that the heart makes as blood flows through it, which may or may not indicate an underlying problem with the heart or the blood vessels around it. There are two main classifications of murmurs: *innocent* and *pathologic*.

An innocent murmur is a sound that may be slightly different from the normal "lub dub" of the heart, but it has no significance. It does not pose any health risk, nor will it affect the child's growth, limit her activity, or require medication. It is merely a sound that the heart makes.

A pathologic murmur, on the other hand, is a sound that the heart makes indicating that there is an underlying problem that needs to be monitored or treated. Fifty percent of all newborns have heart murmurs, but the vast majority are not problematic. The word "murmur" alone may stop your heart, but rest assured that most newborn murmurs are harmless. If your pediatrician has any suspicions that the murmur is not harmless, there are a number of different tests he may order:

- *Pulse oximeter:* A blue-light sensor is taped to your infant's feet or hands to determine how much oxygen she is getting.
- *Four-point blood pressures:* A blood pressure reading is taken on each arm and each leg to make sure the readings are roughly the same, indicating that blood is flowing equally to all parts of the body and there is no obstruction to the flow.
- *Chest X-ray:* A chest X-ray can be helpful to evaluate the size of the heart and make sure that there is no backup of blood flow causing flooding to the lungs.
- *Cardiologist consultation:* An *electrocardiogram* (EKG) will be taken to make sure there is no *arrhythmia*. Or an *echocardiogram* (echo) will be taken to evaluate the structure of the heart and how the blood flows through it.

I realize that these evaluations can cause anxiety for parents, but most are precautionary to confirm a diagnosis. Here are some common diagnoses that should not raise your heart rate if you hear your doctor mention them.

Patent Ductus Arteriosus (PDA)

The *ductus arteriosus* is a vessel that allows oxygen-rich blood from the pregnant mother to travel to the fetus's body. After birth this conduit is no longer needed because oxygenated blood can flow directly from the infant's lungs to her body. An infant's ductus will usually close immediately after birth, but it may take a couple of hours to days. As long as the ductus remains open, a murmur is heard as blood flows through it. This is a very common murmur and not usually a cause for concern. In fact, many pediatricians will wait a day or two, without making an intervention, to see if the murmur disappears on its own, indicating the ductus has closed.

If the ductus does not close, your pediatrician may ask for a cardiologist to obtain an echo to verify the diagnosis. If the ductus does indeed remain open, the infant will have routine visits with the cardiologist every few months until it closes. In full-term infants, this condition will usually not cause any problems or require any special medications. However, in rare cases, the ductus will remain open or be large enough to cause a problem with blood pressure or oxygenation. This is more common in smaller, premature infants. In these cases, the drug indomethacin may be started in the hospital to try to close the ductus, or surgical closure of the ductus will be performed.

Common Sense Bottom Line
If your child has a PDA don't worry. It is very common, and the ductus will most likely close on its own.

Peripheral Pulmonic Stenosis (PPS)

PPS is another murmur common to infants. It occurs as a result of an increase in blood flow to the lungs after birth. Since the infant's blood vessels are too small to accommodate this increase, the turbulence that is created is heard as a murmur. If a murmur consistent with PPS is heard, no further workup is necessary unless the doctor wants to confirm the diagnosis with an echo. A PPS murmur may be heard until the baby is about six months old. After that, the blood vessels to the lungs will have expanded to accommodate the blood flow and the murmur will disappear. If the murmur is still present after six months of age a cardiologist should evaluate it.

Common Sense Bottom Line
Don't worry. Most likely a PPS murmur will go away on its own.

Atrial Septal Defect and Ventriculoseptal Defect

Sometimes infants are born with a "hole in their heart." Although this sounds frightening, it is actually the most common congenital heart defect and is usually self-resolving.

During pregnancy, the heart begins as one chamber that eventually divides into four. Sometimes, when the heart forms, the **55** wall (septum) between the two chambers on the right and the two chambers on the left does not fully fuse, leaving a "hole" between the two sides of the heart. If the hole is between the two upper chambers (atria), it is called an *atrial septal defect* (ASD). If the hole is between the two lower chambers (ventricles), it is called a *ventriculoseptal defect* (VSD). In either case, some of the oxygenated blood from the left side of the heart passes back to the right side in a feedback loop, rather than traveling on to the body. This extra blood flow can be heard as a murmur; however, it usually does not adversely affect your infant.

If your pediatrician detects an ASD or VSD murmur, a cardiologist will be called in to evaluate it with an echo. The good news is that the "hole" usually closes on its own. In most cases, the cardiologist will simply follow up with your baby every few months to make sure that the hole has closed. If the opening is too large to close on its own or is affecting your infant's breathing or eating, a procedure will be performed to close the hole. In healthy infants, this procedure can be delayed until the baby is at least a year old.

Common Sense Bottom Line

Try not to worry. You may have a few extra doctor's appointments, but these "holes" usually close on their own.

Lungs

I remember standing next to my wife during delivery, my heart pounding with anticipation. When our daughter finally made her appearance, she looked like a tiny rag doll, floppy and lifeless. Then, in an instant, she took a breath and came to life: her skin turned pink and she let out the most beautiful cry I had ever heard. I could begin breathing normally again.

Once your child takes her first breath, her breathing is unlikely to be a cause for concern. However, I want to highlight one common newborn breathing issue.

Transient Tachypnea of the Newborn (TTN)

Transient tachypnea of the newborn, as its name suggests, is a fleeting condition caused by fluid in the lungs that results in fast breathing immediately or shortly after birth. It is more common in infants born by cesarean section because they do not get the squeeze of a vaginal birth that helps to expel fluid from the lungs. If fast or labored breathing is detected, a pulse oximeter is used to make sure the baby is receiving enough oxygen. If she is, she will simply be watched closely. Usually the fluid is resorbed into the body within a few hours or, rarely, in a couple of days, but some infants may need oxygen during this time to help them breath more easily. In order to verify the diagnosis of TTN and to rule out other possible conditions, a chest X-ray may be ordered.

Common Sense Bottom Line

Supportive measures will be taken until her breathing improves. Then, once it's gone, it's gone.

Chest

A Training Bra Already?

Some infants—female and male—are born with breast buds. These form when maternal estrogen is transferred to the fetus. One breast may be much bigger than the other or both may be enlarged. You may feel a firm, mobile, pea-sized lump under the nipple, which is a normal breast bud. Or you may see the breasts change in size for weeks to months after birth, especially if Mom is breastfeeding. You may even notice that if you squeeze your baby's nipple gently, milk is expressed. Don't be alarmed. Breast buds and lactation are normal, even in boys, and will go away on their own, usually fairly quickly. However, if your child's breasts are red, swollen, or painful, notify your doctor; this may be a sign of infection.

57

An Olive-Sized Bump

Your infant may have a small, round, firm olive-sized structure protruding from the middle of her chest. This bump is actually a small bone that eventually fuses to make up the sternum or breast plate. As your child grows, her skin will become thicker and less transparent, hiding the sternum from view. In the meantime just ignore it.

Umbilicus (Belly Button)

Shortly after your baby's birth, the obstetrician places two clamps on the umbilical cord and then asks Dad to cut it. Your infant is left with a small remnant of her lifeline attached to her stomach. Now what? How do you take care of it? When will it fall off? Will she have an "inny" or an "outy"? These are all important questions, so what follows is everything you need to know about your child's umbilical cord and belly button.

Does She Have an "Inny" or an "Outy"?

You spend nine months wishing for a healthy child. Then, after the birth, once you know that everything is okay, the vanity kicks in. Whose nose does she have? Will her eyes remain blue? Does she have an "inny" or an "outy"? Whether your child's belly button protrudes or not is mostly luck of the draw. We do not know what produces one or the other, or why 90 percent of people have an "inny."

Sometimes the belly button will look like an "outy," especially when she cries or bears down to poop or pass gas. In fact, this is usually not an "outy" but rather an *umbilical hernia*, which is very common in infants. A hernia is just a hole in the muscle, in this case the abdominal muscle. As your child's abdominal musculature grows thicker and stronger, it usually closes the hole and resolves the hernia. Most umbilical hernias resolve on their own within the first year of life, but some may take several years.

Common Sense Bottom Line

There's no reason to repair an umbilical hernia unless it doesn't close on its own or causes cosmetic concerns to your child later on. As for "inny" or "outy"—makes no difference.

Waiting for the Cord to Fall Off

When you leave the hospital with your newborn, the umbilical cord stump will look hard, shriveled, and black. It usually falls off within two to four weeks. In the meantime, sponge bathe your child in order to keep the cord dry and facilitate its falling off. If you do get it wet, don't worry; it will not hurt your infant, it may just take a little longer to fall off. Remember to spot clean the cord if it becomes soiled with poop.

When the cord falls off, there may be a little blood as it separates. Like any scab that detaches from the body, this is normal. If the area is actively bleeding, notify your pediatrician. There may also be some thick yellow mucus when the cord separates. Although the mucus is as thick as vanilla pudding and smells awful, it's perfectly normal and not an indication of infection. You can dab it gently with dry gauze or leave it alone. Either way, it will crust over and dry up in a couple of days. At that time, you can submerge her belly button in water and bathe your child normally.

A Granu-What?

Sometimes when the cord falls off there is a pink, fleshy remnant that looks like a little ball protruding from the center of the belly button. This is called an *umbilical granuloma*. It is a remnant of the umbilical cord that did not fully fall off. Your pediatrician can apply silver nitrate on the granuloma, which helps it dry up, scab over, and fall off. This does not hurt your child in any way because the silver nitrate only reacts with the wet coating over the granuloma.

Genitalia

Whether you are having a boy or a girl, you should be aware of what you will find under the diaper.

Does Size Really Matter?

Every father waits anxiously for his son's exam under the diaper. Of course, he only cares about one thing: size. I usually do not comment on the size of a baby's penis; however, one child I examined was particularly well endowed. I turned to the parents and commented that their child's penis size was impressive. The dad immediately stood up straight, lifted his shoulders, and stuck out his chest in jubilation. A big grin appeared on his face. I then said, "It is interesting to note that penis size usually comes from Mom's side of the family." I paused. Mom started to giggle. Dad's posture deflated as he looked at me skeptically. When I told him I was kidding he began to laugh and gave a deep sigh of relief.

In general, you should not be concerned about the size of your son's penis. Many infants have penises that appear very small because of the area above the penis, called the *suprapubic fat pad*. The plumper the infant, the larger the fat pad that hides the penis, a condition I call the "peek-a-boo penis." This does not mean that your child's penis is small. As he gets older the fat pad thins out and the penis will pop out.

Common Sense Bottom Line
Size doesn't matter.

It Lights Up Like a Jack-o'-lantern

Parents are sometimes shocked to find how large, pendulous, and dark their son's scrotum is. This is all very normal. The scrotum may look very full and firm, as if it's filled with water. Actually, it is full of fluid. Males are often born with fluid around their testicles called a hydrocele. If you shine a light under your son's scrotum, the sac will light up like a jack-o'-lantern because the fluid transilluminates. This fluid doesn't hurt or affect your son's future libido. It will usually be resorbed into the body by the time he's a year old, if not sooner. If the fluid does not resolve by age one, a urologist should evaluate your child. At that time, a simple procedure can be performed to fix the problem.

Common Sense Bottom Line
Fluid around the testicles is normal until age one. If it persists beyond that time, have your baby evaluated by a urologist.

Circumcision Care

After your infant son's circumcision, the head of his penis will look red and raw. Follow this regimen after every diaper change:

1. *Gently pull back the skin at the base of the penis and clean around the head, using soap and water or baby wipes.* By going through this process, you'll help to prevent the normal skin of the shaft from reattaching over the head of the penis, a condition called *penile adhesion.* If this does occur, however, the shaft can be separated from the head of the penis over time by gently pulling back the skin or, in more severe cases, by using a steroid cream or surgical separation.

2. *Place a piece of gauze with Vaseline or antibacterial ointment over the penis to prevent the healing skin from sticking to the diaper.* Continue this routine until the head of the penis no longer looks irritated, which may take up to one week. As the penis heals, the healing skin may look yellow and crusty. This is not a cause for concern but part of the normal healing process.

3. *When the penis heals don't be surprised if the head of the penis, which resembles a mushroom, has a bluish hue.* Then there will be a red or pink transition area (this is where the foreskin was removed) leading to the normal skin-colored shaft.

You may also notice that your baby's penis secretes a malodorous, white, creamy substance called *smegma.* This may appear along the ridge of the head of the penis, or in what looks like white-headed pimples along the penile shaft. These are normal and will resolve spontaneously, or the white heads will open, at which point you can clean them with a washcloth, soap, and water.

Common Sense Bottom Line
Keep it clean! Make sure your infant's circumcised penis receives proper hygiene.

Uncircumcised Care
Unlike an infant's circumcised penis, an uncircumcised penis appears uniform along its length, leading to a more pointed tip resembling an ear of corn with the husk on it. Uncircumcised males

actually need less maintenance early on because the foreskin will not retract. Parents should, however, gently attempt to retract the foreskin until you reach resistance, and clean any white discharge that is expressed. Over the course of several years, the foreskin will eventually retract fully over the head of the penis.

Common Sense Bottom Line
An infant's uncircumcised penis needs proper hygiene, too!

A Little Off-Center
When you look at your son's penis, the opening to the urethra should be at the tip of the penis. If the hole is a little off-center, that is still normal, but if the hole is on the side of the penis or further down toward the shaft, then it should be evaluated by a urologist. In the meantime, hold off on the circumcision until it is evaluated. The off-center urethral opening is called *hypospadius*, or *epispadius*, depending on the location of the hole, and may require surgical intervention.

Common Sense Bottom Line
An off-center urethral opening is not very common, and chances are there's nothing to worry about. If the opening is dramatically off-center, have your son evaluated by a urologist.

Undescended Testicles
Most males are born with both testicles descended from the abdomen, but don't be alarmed if your son's scrotum looks or feels empty on one side. Sometimes one or both of the testicles are not fully descended, a condition called *cryptorchidism*. This is more common in premature infants because they're born before the testicles have fully come down. If your baby has one or two undescended testicles, don't worry. It doesn't mean that he has insufficient testosterone. It usually just means he needs more time. More than 80 percent of

males' testicles descend by the time they're a year old; however, if your baby's testicles don't descend by nine to twelve months of age, referral to a urologist is warranted.

Common Sense Bottom Line

Give them time to descend—and don't worry! If his testicles are still unde- scended after nine to twelve months, have your son seen by a urologist.

Baby Girl Vaginal Hygiene

In baby girls, it is normal for the labia to look swollen and for there to be vaginal discharge. This discharge may be yellow, white, green, gray, or bloody, like a small period. This is all due to Mom's hor- mones and is perfectly normal. When you change your daughter's diaper, don't be afraid to spread the labia and wipe out the poop and discharge with soap and water or baby wipes. Do your best to keep her clean, but don't worry if you don't get every nook and cranny. Do make sure to wipe baby girls from front to back to pre- vent bacteria from getting into the vagina.

Pink Stain in the Diaper

It's normal during the first week of your baby's life to see a pink stain in her diaper. This is not blood but *uric acid crystals* that form when an infant's urine is concentrated. This is not harmful to the infant and is common in a baby's first few days, until Mom's breast milk comes in. As the volume of her intake increases, the pink stain will disappear.

Common Sense Bottom Line

Don't panic—it's not blood. The pink will vanish once she guzzles more milk. If it persists, speak to your pediatrician to make sure your infant is receiving adequate hydration.

Skin

You may be surprised by the multitude of rashes your child develops as a newborn, but most are normal and will never cause any problems.

She's Molting

Most newborns have dry, peeling skin, especially on their hands and feet—you would, too, if you had just spent nine months in water. The peeling is normal, and if you leave it alone it will go away on its own; however, you can use a moisturizing cream on her body and face to speed up the process.

You may also notice little red bumps on her skin, and a texture that's dry and rough like sandpaper. This can also be treated with moisturizing cream. Remember, bathing your child frequently can cause dryness so a moisturizing massage after baths is recommended.

Common Sense Bottom Line
Dry skin is common among new babies. Don't worry—moisturize!

What's That Blue Line Between Her Eyes?

You may notice a blue line on your baby's forehead or between her eyes and wonder if it's a birthmark. Usually what you are seeing is a vein. Because infants have thinner, more translucent skin, the vein is more noticeable. As their skin gets darker and thicker, you won't notice it anymore.

Flea Bites?

Despite its horrible-sounding name, *erythema toxicum* is an absolutely normal newborn rash. We don't know what causes it, but it's harmless. It looks like little flea bites with a red bump in the center surrounded by a red blotchy ring. This rash may appear soon after delivery and come and go for several weeks, appearing on any part of the body from head to toe. It's not painful or itchy and it won't scar.

Little Whiteheads

Another common newborn rash looks like little whiteheads, and it can appear anywhere on the body. As the whiteheads break, they leave an area of peeling skin that may be slightly darker at the center. This rash, which is called *transient neonatal pustular melanosis,* may be present at birth and can last for several weeks to a few months.

Even Tinier Whiteheads

Another common rash that's usually found on an infant's nose and forehead looks like pinhead-sized whiteheads called *milia.* No need for facials, they'll clear up on their own.

Neonatal Acne

Neonatal acne may look worse than a teenager's. Your infant may have red bumps and whiteheads all over her face, chest, and back caused by maternal hormones. Neonatal acne may come and go for months, but no treatment is necessary and there's no risk of scarring. *Do not* use medications such as benzoyl peroxide or Proactive—these are not intended for babies and are unnecessary. Simply wash your baby's skin with a soft soap and water.

Common Sense Bottom Line

Baby acne bothers you more than it bothers her. Hit the soap and water and ditch the vanity.

Mongolian Spots

Mongolian spots are flat blue blotches that look like bruises and are most common on an infant's back and buttocks, though they may appear anywhere on her body. They're more common in certain ethnic groups, especially Asians and African Americans. The spots may fade over time or become less noticeable as the skin gets thicker and darker. Either way, they'll never cause your baby any problems.

Common Sense Bottom Line

They're not bruises—ignore them.

Red Splotchy Stork's Kisses

The flat, red splotches that often appear on the eyelids (where they look like red eye shadow), mid-forehead, or nape of the neck are known as stork's kisses. These birthmarks are made of blood vessels, and become redder when your child cries or strains to poop. They usually fade or disappear with time, and will never cause a problem.

> ### Daddy vs. Doctor—The Stork's Kiss
>
> During my wife's entire pregnancy, whenever anyone asked if I wanted a boy or a girl, I would reply, "It doesn't matter—just healthy." Then, as soon as she was born and I realized she was healthy, vanity kicked in. Did she have my nose or my wife's? Would she keep her blue eyes? Would all of her hair fall out? Did she have any birthmarks?
>
> She did. She had a stork's kiss on her left upper eyelid. Surprisingly, though, it never bothered us. If it went away, great. If it didn't, who cares? She was healthy and perfect no matter what.
>
> There are plenty of things to worry about in life and this was just not one of them.

Hemangioma

Hemangiomas are a common vascular birthmark. There are two types: *strawberry* and *cavernous*. Strawberry hemangiomas are red, raised blotches that may feel warm to the touch. The red color is due to an accumulation of blood vessels on the top of the skin. Cavernous hemangiomas are usually bluish, because the blood vessels are *under* the skin, and feel doughy. Both types are the result of blood vessel growth hormones that circulate in the baby's body during the first year of life. After the first year, they'll begin to recede and disappear, which may take five to seven years.

Intervention is only needed if the birthmark is in a location where it may cause an obstruction (such as the ear, mouth, nose, or eyes) or if the hemangioma is large and bleeds. In these cases oral steroids or laser treatment can be administered to try to reduce the size.

Common Sense Bottom Line
They may not be beautiful, but they're temporary and won't cause any harm.

Jaundice

Jaundice describes the yellow color of the skin caused by an accumulation of *bilirubin*, the breakdown product of hemoglobin, which makes up our red blood cells. Jaundice always starts on the face and moves down the body. The more yellow the infant, the more severe the jaundice.

Jaundice is caused by either an overproduction of bilirubin or an obstruction in its excretion. The obstruction may occur anywhere in the pathway between production, processing in the liver, and excretion in the stool and urine. More than 50 percent of infants develop jaundice, but luckily, most have only mild jaundice and require no treatment. If jaundice is detected, your doctor will look at the infant's skin daily to see if the color is getting better or order blood tests to monitor the level of bilirubin. The concern is due to a rare condition called kernicterus, in which high levels of bilirubin may damage the brain. Depending on the level of bilirubin, your doctor will discuss possible causes and treatment options.

The causes of jaundice can be distinguished by the level of bilirubin, how old the child was when the jaundice began, and supporting blood work.

The most common causes of jaundice are:

Healthy Baby (Physiologic) Jaundice (Two to Three Days Old)

In healthy baby jaundice, you'll notice the yellow color when your baby is around two to three days old. There are two contributors to this type of jaundice:

1. Slight dehydration in the first couple of days of life because of Mom's breast milk not coming in yet (resulting in a higher concentration of bilirubin in the baby's blood);
2. Inefficiency of the newborn's liver, which is common because it takes a few days for the liver to "rev up" and start processing bilirubin for excretion.

Fortunately, right around the time your child starts to turn yellow, Mom's milk comes in to flush out her system and the liver

69

becomes more efficient and starts pushing the bilirubin out of the body in the stool and urine. The jaundice will then begin to resolve over the next couple of days to a week.

Breastfeeding Jaundice (Four to Seven Days Old)

Another common jaundice in the newborn is breastfeeding jaundice, which usually begins when the infant is around four to seven days old. Contrary to its name, this type of jaundice occurs because Mom's breast milk has not fully come in yet and the baby is dehydrated, resulting in a higher concentration of bilirubin in her blood. The infant may be having less stool and urine output, leading to less excretion of bilirubin, which can then exacerbate the jaundice.

If this type of jaundice is suspected, your baby's diet will be supplemented with either pumped breast milk or formula until the jaundice improves. Strategies to increase breast milk supply will be employed as well. In some situations, the infant may need to sleep under special *bilirubin lights* at home or in the hospital until supplementation can adequately diminish the jaundice.

Breast Milk Jaundice (Seven to Ten Days Old)

Although it sounds similar to breastfeeding jaundice, breast milk jaundice usually appears when the infant is around seven to ten days old and is caused by a particular enzyme found in breast milk that increases the amount of bilirubin in the blood. This type of jaundice is not harmful, but if there is a question as to the cause of the jaundice, a definitive diagnosis can be made by stopping breastfeeding for a couple of days to see if the bilirubin level decreases. If it does, then it is breast milk jaundice, and there's nothing to worry about.

Blood Incompatibilities

A less common cause of newborn jaundice that may need treatment is a blood incompatibility, and the two most common are Rh and ABO incompatibility.

Rh Incompatibility (First Twenty-four Hours of Life)
Blood type is designated by a letter (A, B, O, or AB) followed by a positive or negative sign. The positive or negative portion of the blood

type is called the Rh factor. If a mother is Rh negative and her first child is Rh positive, the mother's body will produce antibodies against the positive blood type when she is exposed to that child's blood during delivery. These antibodies will not affect this first child, because she will be born before the antibodies are fully produced. However, if Mom has a second child with a positive Rh, her antibodies will attack the infant's red blood cells, causing the breakdown of red blood cells and jaundice. This type of jaundice occurs in the first twenty-four hours of life, is usually severe, and can be life-threatening. Treatment is initiated immediately and the infant will be monitored closely.

Due to the possibility of an infant's severe reaction, mothers with a negative Rh receive RhoGAM at twenty-eight weeks gestation and then again shortly after delivery during each pregnancy. RhoGAM contains antibodies that block the maternal antibodies so they cannot attack the infant.

ABO Incompatibility

If the mother is blood type O and the baby is either an A or B blood type, a reaction similar to Rh incompatibility may occur, but not as severely. Fortunately, this reaction does not occur with every mother and child with these blood types, but, if jaundice is noted in a child whose mother is blood type O, the child's blood type will be tested to see if there is a reaction. Depending on the severity of the jaundice, treatment may be initiated or the child will simply be monitored.

Other Causes of Jaundice

There are many other causes of jaundice, including infections, liver disease, metabolic disorders, and hypothyroidism. Fortunately, they are not common and you should not worry about them.

Treatment

The vast majority of infants with jaundice will not require any treatment. However, if your doctor determines that your child's bilirubin level has risen to a significant level, he will recommend *phototherapy,* or, in severe cases (and much less common), an *exchange transfusion.*

Phototherapy works by shining light on the skin, thus degrading the bilirubin so it can be excreted from the body. Infants will often be placed on a *bilirubin blanket* (a blanket of lights) as well as under a lamp, so that her back and front are exposed simultaneously. Bilirubin lights are safe and effective, but it's important that the infant wear protective eyewear and receive adequate fluids to prevent dehydration.

An exchange transfusion removes the blood, with the high level of bilirubin, and replaces it with a donor's blood whose bilirubin levels are normal. The net effect is to dilute the high concentration of bilirubin in the infant and decrease the level of jaundice.

Common Sense Bottom Line

Jaundice is common and can usually be treated easily. In most cases, all that is needed is to wait and watch.

Healthy baby jaundice: *No special tests or treatment is usually needed—nothing to worry about.*

Breastfeeding jaundice: *Breast milk is taking too long to come in, so pumped breast milk or formula may be required. Baby may be placed under lights in some circumstances. Nothing to worry about.*

Breast milk jaundice: *Caused by an enzyme in Mom's milk—nothing to worry about.*

Blood incompatibility jaundice: *Baby will be monitored more closely and a treatment may be suggested.*

Extremities

Your pediatrician will check your baby's extremities to see that she has ten fingers, ten toes, good blood flow to the extremities, and normal skin color. However, you may have other concerns.

Smurftastic

Believe it or not, it's common for your baby's hands and feet to look blue. This is because of an infant's immature circulatory system, and the blueness may be exacerbated by temperature or positioning. If her hands and feet feel cold, rub them gently to warm them up and they'll turn pink again. You may notice that her legs turn blue if she's in a carrier with her legs dangling. This is due to compression of the circulation, which you can remedy simply by changing her position.

Common Sense Bottom Line
Blue hands and feet are normal—they may just need warming up or repositioning.

Why Are Her Hands and Feet So Sweaty?

Babies typically have sweaty hands and feet. This will not affect their dating life, nor does it mean they'll become a sweaty adult. Unless your infant has a fever, there's nothing to worry about.

Muscle Tone, Strength, and Reflexes

Every child is born with innate reflexes that will later disappear. They are normal and here's how you can test your baby's reflexes.

Startle Reflex

You don't have to jump out of the closet to elicit this reflex. Lay your child on her back and place one of your fingers in the palm of each of her hands until she grasps it. Gently pull up until you break her grasp. You'll notice that she jumps a little and that her arms shake and hug the air. She may do this many times a day, even out of a dead sleep. This is a normal newborn reflex.

Toe Curl Reflex (Babinski Reflex)

If you give your significant other a foot massage, gently rubbing the bottom of his foot from top to bottom, his toes will curl down. When you try it on your newborn, her toes will curl up instead. This toe curl (*Babinski*) reflex is present until one year of age, at which time the toes start curling down to help grasp the floor while walking.

Suck Reflex

The suck reflex is obviously crucial. It is both comforting for your newborn and necessary for feeding. Stick your finger in her mouth and bend it until you touch the roof of her mouth. This stimulates a baby's suck reflex.

Eye-blinking Reflex (Glabellar Reflex)

Gently tap the middle of your baby's forehead. Every time you tap she will blink her eyes. Now try it on a friend. He may blink the first couple of times, but not after that.

Rooting Reflex

Gently tickle one cheek. Notice the corner of your baby's mouth closest to that cheek start to move toward your stroking. This reflex causes your child to naturally move her mouth to a prospective food source—so that when the nipple touches her cheek she will move her mouth to find it.

Grasp Reflex

Place your finger in the palm of your baby's hand and she will grab it tightly. Now try and break her kung-fu grip.

Stepping Reflex

Hold your infant upright by carrying her under her arms and supporting her head and neck. Let her feet touch the floor and watch as she starts "walking." This doesn't mean she is ready to actually walk, but it is a neat trick.

Fencing Reflex

I like to call this the Heisman reflex. Lay your baby on her back and gently turn her head to one side. The arm on the opposite side will flex or bend at the elbow as if she is showing you her muscles, and the arm she is facing will extend as if she is posing for the Heisman.

Galant Reflex

Place your infant on her stomach and gently stroke her back from her neck down the side of the spinal column toward her butt. If you stroke to the right of the spinal cord she will bend her body in that direction. If you stroke to the left she will bend left. Now play some music and do a little dance.

Baby Quirks

Soon after your infant is born you are going to witness some pretty strange things, which I like to refer to as baby quirks. Infants shake and hug the air like tiny tribal dancers. Their legs shiver and their lower lips and chins quiver like mini-Elvis impersonators. They sneeze when they're not sick; hiccup like crazy; breathe fast, then slow, then fast again; and finally, they do an amazing impression of Darth Vader.

So here are some typical baby quirks that may seem unusual or scary, but are absolutely nothing to worry about.

The King

Though she won't be dancing to "Jailhouse Rock," you may notice your newborn's legs shake and lower lip and chin quiver for no reason. These tremors only last a couple of seconds and are simply the result of her immature nervous system. In a few months, her Elvis impersonations will vanish. If she jumps and hugs the air with arms outstretched and shakes gently, remember that this is the normal newborn startle reflex, which will lessen by four to six months.

Sneezy

Sneezy of the Seven Dwarfs doesn't hold a candle to many newborns, who sneeze constantly. But there's nothing to worry about since newborn sneezing has nothing to do with allergies or sickness; it's simply how they expel dust and air.

Hiccups

How can you make an infant stop hiccupping?

1. Hide behind her bassinet and scare her when she wakes up from a nap.

2. Have her hold her breath for ten seconds.

3. Tell her to chug breast milk really quickly.

4. None of the above.

Babies hiccup because they are always swallowing air, and although their whole body may convulse with each hiccup, it doesn't bother them—don't let it bother you.

On Again/Off Again Breathing

Most adults breathe at a constant, even rate. Infants, on the other hand, may breathe very fast, pause, then take a deep breath. This is called *periodic breathing*. The first time you see your child pause during her breathing cycle you may hold your own breath in worry and anticipation. Do not worry. This is normal newborn breathing, so breathe easy.

Baby Darth

With their loud deep breathing, most infants do a pretty good impression of Darth Vader. That's because they tend to be nasal breathers. Whereas most adults are adept at breathing through their mouth, infants prefer to breathe through their nose, which allows them to feed and breathe comfortably at the same time.

There are several reasons your infant may sound congested. First, every infant has small nasal passages. On top of that, infants spend most of their time on their backs, so their airways narrow a little with gravity. Second, feeding is strenuous exercise, and they're trying to force as much air through their small airways as possible. Finally, when infants spit up, some of the milk ends up in the upper airways, leaving less space for the air to pass through and creating a more congested sound. Makes sense, right?

All of this is normal, but if your child seems uncomfortable because of congestion, elevate the head of her bed 45 degrees or run a cool mist vaporizer in the room to loosen up nasal secretions and help her breathe easier. You can also use a bulb suction and saline drops to help remove any pesky mucus blocking the airway. But don't be overzealous.

Common Sense Bottom Line

If she sounds like Darth Vader but nothing's bothering her, ignore it. If you see something, and that something is bothering her, suck it out . . . and may the Force be with you.

Each of these "baby quirks" are weird and wacky, but nothing to worry about—so don't!

CHAPTER 4

EAT

Breast, Bottle, and Beyond

· ·

I t seems that nearly every new mom and dad is stressed out about why to breastfeed, how to breastfeed, when to breastfeed, where to breastfeed, and at what point it's okay to stop breastfeeding. Breastfeeding worries have parents so frenzied that conversations concerning this topic begin to sound like a Three Stooges skit. A simple biological function that women throughout the world have been performing from day one has become a source of very high anxiety. So my job in this chapter is to de-stress you when it comes to all things related to breastfeeding—and beyond, like bottles, formula, and the light at the end of the tunnel: introducing solid foods.

My Common Sense Parenting bottom line here is that you need to worry less about the rigid rules and schedules surrounding what and how and when your baby eats, and focus instead on simply satisfying her basic needs, while at the same time making life more enjoyable and sane for everyone in your family. In this chapter, we'll touch all the major bases of breastfeeding, bottle feeding, formula—and beyond, including:

- Benefits of breast milk
- Scheduled versus on-demand feeding
- Spit-up
- Introducing the bottle

- Breast pumps
- Nipple selection
- Maternal diet and allergies
- Balancing breast milk and formula
- Types of formula
- How and when to stop breastfeeding

And, yes, there is a beyond:

- Introducing solid foods

Breastfeeding Basics

Is It Milk Yet?—Transitioning from Colostrum to Breast Milk

In the first few days following your baby's birth, if you're the mom you'll produce *colostrum,* a high-mineral shake with all the nutrients your infant needs. But there won't be much of it, so your baby may want to feed more frequently. She may also lose up to 10 percent of her weight in the first week. In general, there's no need to worry about this. If she loses too much or the milk is taking longer to come in, you and your pediatrician will discuss whether or not supplementing with formula is necessary. Usually, when the baby is around three to five days old, the breast milk begins to come in.

You'll know that breast milk is coming in from several signs. First, your breasts will feel fuller (more "engorged") and you may be able to express white breast milk from the nipple. During feeding, you may hear your child gulp or swallow and see milk in or around her mouth when she's done. You'll also notice that her poop will change color, from black to a transitional green to a watery mustard yellow. And by the time she's two weeks old, she'll regain her birth weight.

Got Milk?—The Advantages of Breast Milk

Breastfeeding has been shown to be beneficial to both the infant and the mother. For the infant, breast milk decreases the incidence of:

- diarrhea
- lower respiratory infections
- ear infections
- bacteria in the blood and bacterial meningitis
- urinary tract infections
- infection of the intestine

Some studies have also shown that breast milk may decrease the risk of:

- SIDS
- allergic diseases and allergic sensitivity of the skin
- ulcerative colitis and Crohn's disease
- insulin-dependent diabetes mellitus

And breast milk may even enhance cognitive function. (Yes, Albert Einstein was reportedly breastfed for the first year of his life.)

For the mother, breastfeeding is beneficial because it:

- creates a bond between mother and child
- increases oxytocin, resulting in less postpartum bleeding
- leads to earlier return to prepregnancy weight
- improves bone mineralization
- decreases risk of ovarian cancer
- decreases risk of premenopausal breast cancer

There are also convenience considerations and economic benefits to breastfeeding, including zero food preparation time, zero money spent on infant formula, and a completely portable food supply.

The Milk Stops Here—When Not to Breastfeed

There are, however, a number of situations in which mothers should *not* breastfeed. These include:

- if you use illicit drugs
- if you are infected with HIV

- if you have active tuberculosis
- if you are on chemotherapy medications
- if you are undergoing radiation therapy
- if your infant has a rare genetic disorder called *galactosemia* (inability to break down galactose, a component of lactose)

Can I Breastfeed If I'm Sick?

In a word: yes. Actually, breast milk is the best thing for your baby even when you're sick, because she is receiving your antibodies to help prevent infection.

Most over-the-counter and common prescription medications are safe to use during breastfeeding. It's also safe to breastfeed if you have a cold or flu. Several precautions do apply, though: if you're sick and not eating well, it may affect your breast milk supply, so make sure you drink plenty of liquids. Also, this may be stating the obvious, but don't cough or sneeze in your infant's face, and make sure to wash your hands well.

Medications Safe for Use by Breastfeeding Mothers

Acyclovir
Advil (ibuprofen)
Albuterol
Allopurinol
Amoxicillin
Ampicillin
Ancef (cefazolin)
Atrovent
Augmenin
Bactrim/Septra (after two months old)
Bactroban (mupirocin)
Barium
Benadryl (diphenhydramine)
Biaxin (clarithromycin)
Ceftin (cefuroxime)

Cefzil (cefprozil)
Ciprofloxacin
Claritin (loratidine)
Colace (docusate)
Coumadin (warfarin)
Dextromethorphan
Diflucan (fluconazole)
Domperidone
Elimite (permethrin)
Erythromycin
Fluoride
Gentamicin
Heparin
Hydrocortisone Cream
Imitrex (sumatriptan)
Imodium (loperamide)

81

Insulin
Kaopectate
Keflex (cephalexin)
Maalox
Macrobid/Macrodantin
    (nitrofurantoin)
Milk of Magnesia
Monistat (miconazole)
Motrin (ibuprofen)
Nix (permethrin)
Nystatin
Omnicef (cefdinir)
Pepcid (famotidine)
Robitussin (guaifenesin)

Rocephin (ceftriaxone)
Scopolamine Patch
Suprax (cefixime)
Synthroid (levothyroxine)
Tagamet (cimetidine)
Tylenol (acetaminophen)
Valtrex (valacycolvir)
Xopenex (levalbuterol)
Zantac (ranitidine)
Zithromax (azithromycin)
Zyrtec (ceirizine)
Over-the-counter cough/
    cold/sore throat
    remedies

As for herbal supplements, many have not been studied and as a result have not been approved by the FDA. Their effect on nursing babies is unknown.

Antidepressants (Prozac, Zoloft, Paxil) are in a category in which there are either no controlled studies in breastfeeding women or controlled studies show only minimal nonthreatening adverse effects. Because there are not enough studies to deem them "safe," each parent must weigh whether the potential benefit of taking the medication justifies the potential risk to the baby.

What Should I Eat While I'm Breastfeeding?

A common worry is that Mom's diet will make the baby fussy or gassy, or cause an allergic reaction. My overall advice is that you should eat anything you want. If you want sushi, have some. If you crave a cheeseburger with onions, indulge. If you want to celebrate with a glass of wine or beer, feel free. Even peanut butter is fine. Most children are not allergic to anything, and studies on the diets of breastfeeding moms and their affect on infant allergies are not conclusive.

With that said, if you find that when you eat a specific food and your child is more gassy or fussy after breastfeeding, eliminate that food. If you're not sure which food your baby is reacting to, try the following elimination diet.

- Eliminate one food for three to four days and see if your child's demeanor after feeding improves.
- The most common problem foods in maternal diets are dairy, citrus, and eggs. Start by eliminating dairy for three to four days and see if it makes a difference. When you eliminate dairy also eliminate soy, because 10 to 15 percent of people who are allergic to the cow's milk protein in dairy are also allergic to soy protein.
- If you notice an improvement in your child's reaction to breastfeeding, you've likely found the problem. This doesn't mean you have to abstain from that particular food. In fact, slowly reintroduce that food back into your diet and you may find a threshold where your infant is not affected. For instance, if you have a glass of milk, your child might be fine, but if you have a glass of milk, a yogurt, a bowl of ice cream, and some cheese, she's super fussy and gassy.
- If you don't notice a difference with the elimination of a certain food, reintroduce it and eliminate something else.
- If you don't find the culprit after dairy, citrus, and eggs are eliminated, try eliminating tomatoes, green vegetables, spicy food, or caffeine.

Common Sense Bottom Line
Eat what appeals to you in moderation (with an emphasis on healthy, nutritional foods), and drink plenty of liquids. If your child seems to be reacting adversely to your diet, eliminate one food at a time to pinpoint the problem food.

If I Drink Alcohol, Should I Pump and Dump?

I've had new moms tell me that if they go out for dinner and have a glass of wine, they feel they should come home and "pump and dump" their breast milk so that it doesn't get into their baby's system. There is no need to do this. Doctors don't know exactly how much alcohol gets into the milk, but it is a very small amount, if any, and should not cause problems. With that said, you definitely shouldn't go on a drinking binge while you're nursing. But do feel free to eat and drink whatever you want within moderation. If you are concerned about your baby getting too much alcohol in your breast milk, breastfeed right before you have a drink to maximize the time between the alcohol and the next feeding.

Common Sense Bottom Line
It's fine to have an occasional glass of wine or beer. However, if you notice that your child is a little sleepier or feeding poorly after you've had alcohol to drink, stop.

Scheduled versus On-Demand Feeding

When's Dinner?
I remember as a kid running into my house, famished after playing outside, and yelling, "When's dinner?" As a parent, you'll be hearing that question for the next eighteen years or so. At this point, it'll be asked in the form of your infant's cry—every few hours.

Remember the numbers two and four because they will provide the answers to most of your feeding questions. *For the first two to four months of your baby's life, she'll normally want to feed every two to four hours. And when she takes a bottle, she'll take about two to four ounces.*

Some parents keep journals of their infant's feeding schedule, including: what time she fed, how long she fed, where she fed, how many wet diapers, how many poopy diapers, outside temperature, wind velocity, latitude, longitude . . . you name it. Which begs the question: Do you really need to schedule your child's feedings or can you assume that she will let you know when she's hungry? It's up to you to choose the method that works best for you and your baby, but feeding on demand makes the most sense to me. If you do choose to put your child on a schedule, such as nine a.m., twelve p.m., three p.m., six p.m., nine p.m., that's fine. But you'll need to be willing to wake your child to feed her if she's sleeping during one of her designated feeding times—and why would you ever want to wake a sleeping baby?

On the other hand, if you feed her on demand, she'll fall into her own schedule of eating, generally ranging between every two to every four hours. And when she's asleep, you can let her sleep. I recommend *not* waking her up at night once your milk is in. During the day, on the other hand, I would never let a baby sleep more than four hours for the obvious reason that if she sleeps longer stretches during the day, she and you are going to be up more at night.

But just because she's awake more hours during the day doesn't mean she won't wake you up at night when she's hungry. If your child is hungry, she will let you know—no matter what time it is. No need to worry about a healthy infant starving herself by sleeping when she should be eating. She'll wake up, and she'll let you know it's time for a meal. On the other hand, if she gives you the gift of a four-, six-, or even eight-hour stretch of sleep at night— fantastic! But don't tell any new parents you know, because you'll end up with a lot of jealous friends.

If you're feeding on demand but your child is not gaining weight, or if your baby is premature, your pediatrician may ask you to feed her more frequently. In general, though, follow your baby's cues. Feed her regularly during the day and at night if she awakens and is hungry.

Common Sense Bottom Line
Feed on demand, expect to be awakened at night . . . but don't wake a sleeping baby!

Common Sense Exception to the Bottom Line: Feeding Twins
With twins, I recommend "scheduling" the feedings in the sense that the baby who wakes up first becomes the "decider." When one baby wakes up hungry, wake up the other baby so that you can feed them both at roughly the same time. Otherwise the feedings are going to be staggered every hour and you'll never get any sleep.

Do I Have to Follow the Eight-Twenty-Four Rule?

If you haven't already heard about it, let me introduce you to my so-called eight-twenty-four rule. Some folks say that you need to feed your infant *eight* times per day, *twenty* minutes on each breast, and make sure they receive the *fore*milk and *hind*milk. (Foremilk has a more watery content while hindmilk contains more fat.) Despite their names, hindmilk and foremilk do not flow one after the other, respectively. In fact, breast milk is made continuously, transitioning gradually between the two, and both components are an important part of your infant's nutrition. Interestingly, it appears the amount of fat in breast milk is related to how full or empty the breast is at a given time (a greater proportion of fat when the breast is half full compared to when the breast is fully engorged). And weight gain is simply related to the volume of milk consumed, not its fat content. So much for the foremilk/ hindmilk part of the rule.

As for the precise requirement of eight times a day, twenty minutes on each breast? Forgettaboutit. Your child is the most highly developed parasite on earth. She'll take what she needs when she needs it. Some infants feed for twenty minutes on each breast per feeding, while other infants may take three to five minutes on one breast and get what they need. If she is taking a shorter time on the breast and seems satiated, this is usually a good sign. It means she is strong and efficient and you are producing well. Follow your infant's cues. Don't worry if she doesn't feed eight times a day. Maybe she only feeds six times. Maybe one day she feeds ten times. It all averages out, and if she's gaining weight and happy, she's getting what she needs. Believe me, if you take your baby off your breast when she's still hungry, she'll scream until you give her more. And if you try to force her to eat more when she's full, she'll pull away.

If your baby takes only one breast during a feeding, offer her the other breast the following feeding to help balance your production and minimize your risk of engorgement.

Common Sense Bottom Line

Follow your infant's cues, not a locker combination. If it makes you feel better to keep track of the time of every feeding and the length of time on each breast, go for it. But if your child is feeding every two to four hours when she's awake, appears satiated after the feeding, and is gaining weight, don't worry about the timing or the type of milk your child is receiving.

Is It Okay to Be a Human Pacifier?

It's very common for newborns to want to breastfeed for a couple of minutes, fall asleep on the breast, then feed another few minutes and fall asleep again, especially in the first few days of life. In fact, your infant would be very happy to do this for twenty-four hours a day if you let her. But you don't want your child to use your breast as a pacifier because she'll come to depend on it as the only means of relaxation and falling asleep. So I recommend that you not allow her to spend more than twenty to twenty-five minutes on each breast per feeding. Any longer than that and she won't really be receiving extra nutritional benefit. Also, you'll likely get sore and no longer enjoy the breastfeeding experience.

If your baby seems sleepy when it's time to feed, do what you can to arouse her. Take off her clothes so she can feel your skin-to-skin contact. Change her diaper. Wipe her face with a cool washcloth.

If she begins to fuss less than two hours from the last feeding, try soothing her first before putting her back on the breast. She may just want a little comfort, so try swaddling or holding 87 her, *shhhhhh*-ing her, or using a pacifier. If this works, it means she wasn't hungry but just wanted to be comforted.

Spit-up

Scenes from The Exorcist—Spit-up

Spit-up is a normal part of infancy, and may occur as frequently as every feeding or rarely at all. Even if your child resembles something out of *The Exorcist,* it doesn't mean she needs treatment. I remember one five-month-old who would spit up after every feeding and then start giggling. Her parents thought there must be something wrong with her, but in fact she was perfectly normal.

When it comes to spit-up, I have learned two things:

1. Make sure I never hold an infant over my head with my mouth open.
2. Bring an extra shirt to work.

The most common causes of spitting up include normal gas, overfeeding, and reflux. So let's discuss these one at a time.

Normal Gas

Spitting up after feeding is usually due to a gas bubble accompanied by milk. You may be alarmed by the quantity and forcefulness of the output, but even though it can look like she spit up more then she took in, it is only a small amount. There's no need to refeed her. Sometimes the spit up can be so forceful that it exits both the mouth and nose. Still normal, don't worry.

Common Sense Bottom Line

If your child has been feeding well and gaining weight, don't be alarmed by spit-up. It's gross but normal, so as long as it doesn't bother her, don't let it bother you.

Overfeeding

It is common for infants to take two to four ounces of milk every two to four hours in the first two to four months of life. However, occasionally some bottle-fed infants will take four to six ounces or more during a feed. If your child seems to vomit after taking in larger quantities, consider lowering the amount a little. The quantity your infant receives from the breast is more difficult to assess, but it's impossible to overfeed your infant on the breast.

A child who is overfed may spit up immediately after a feeding or more than one hour later. The spit-up that occurs shortly after feeding is usually watery and thin in consistency, whereas the spit-up an hour later is usually undigested milk that is thick, curdled, and may have a foul odor. The latter usually occurs because your child is lying down or moving about and pushes the excess milk out of the stomach.

Common Sense Bottom Line

Decrease the volume of the bottle feeding or lengthen the interval between feedings and you should see an improvement in the frequency of spitting up.

Reflux

Another reason for spitting up is *gastroesophageal reflux* (GERD), which is very common in both infants and adults (where it is described as heartburn), especially premature infants, because of the poor muscle tone of their digestive system. Instead of the food being held down in the stomach, it passes through to the esophagus and sometimes even out of the mouth or nose. Also, since infants are on their backs most of the time, they don't have the added advantage of gravity to hold the food down. Fortunately, most reflux is not painful.

Typically, reflux occurs fifteen to thirty minutes after a feeding, and it may take place more frequently when the baby is lying down. Your child will probably not be bothered by reflux spit-up, which is why we call these infants "happy spitters." If your child is a "happy spitter," keep her upright at a forty-five-degree angle for at least fifteen minutes after feeding and elevate the head of her bed by putting a blanket or pillow under the mattress or inserting a wedge.

If your baby experiences pain with reflux or is vomiting so much that she is not gaining weight, then you should seek treatment. Less than one-third of infants fall into this category. Since your baby can't describe the pain of heartburn, she will instead arch her back and cry as she is spitting up because the acid hurts as it moves up the esophagus. Infants with painful reflux will take the bottle or breast without a problem, but within thirty minutes after the feeding they will start to get fussy, spit up, arch their back, and stiffen their body in pain. (Arching the back at other times, especially when upset, is not necessarily a sign that your baby has painful reflux.)

There are a number of options, both medical and non-medical, for treating painful reflux:

1. Position your child upright after feedings for at least fifteen minutes in order to hold the milk down.
2. Try elevating the head of her bed when she goes to sleep.
3. If steps 1 and 2 don't work, try thickening the bottle feeds by adding a teaspoon of rice cereal to her milk (make sure that the milk is not too thick to flow from the nipple) or purchase a thickening formula such as Enfamil AR. The thicker the feed, the less likely it will come up.

4. If your child continues to have painful reflux or have problems gaining weight because of the persistent vomiting, one of several medications can be administered, including Zantac and Prevacid. The medication will decrease the acid in the stomach so that even if your child vomits she will not be in pain. It may subsequently decrease the reflux as well.

Common Sense Bottom Line

It doesn't matter if your child spits up with every feeding, as long it doesn't bother her and she is gaining weight. If she's experiencing pain or is vomiting and losing weight, try the treatment options above. Your baby can usually be weaned off medication by one year of age, if not sooner, as she outgrows her reflux.

Projectile Vomiting

Some infants will projectile vomit after feeding. If your baby does this occasionally, there's nothing to worry about. If she does it after *each* feeding, you should notify your pediatrician. It may be a sign of a rare disorder called *pyloric stenosis,* which usually presents around six to eight weeks of age and is caused by a thickening of the muscle around the *pyloric sphincter,* at the exit of the stomach. Your doctor can diagnose pyloric stenosis by ordering a simple abdominal ultrasound.

Spitting Up Blood

If your child has a small streak of blood in her spit-up, but is otherwise acting normal, feeding well, and does not have a fever, don't be alarmed. Check to see if your nipples are cracked or bleeding, as this may be the cause of the blood in your baby's spit-up. Contact your physician if this is the case, as you may have a yeast infection. Or you may simply need to apply a moisturizer such as lanolin cream on your nipples to heal the chapped skin.

If your child has recurrent bouts of blood in her spit-up, as well as fever, poor feeding, abdominal distention, or unusual behavior, contact your pediatrician immediately.

Introducing the Bottle

Human or Plastic?—Introducing the Bottle

Parents often ask me, "When is the right time to offer our baby a bottle?" They're worried that once their child starts the bottle, she might refuse the breast—a dilemma sometimes referred to as "nipple confusion." Let me just say this: I don't believe in nipple confusion. After all, is it really that hard for a baby to tell the difference between Mom's nipple and a bright orange plastic one? Maybe nipple confusion is not confusion at all but rather nipple common sense. If you had the choice between working really hard for breast milk and getting very little or lying back and having someone pour the milk into your mouth, which would you choose?

I recommend waiting until your infant is at least two weeks old, if possible, to introduce a bottle. This will allow your infant to firmly establish her proficiency at breastfeeding. You may hear from others that you should wait a month or six weeks, and you are more than welcome to do so, but you *can* introduce a bottle earlier. Your baby will have no problem going back and forth between the two. Offer a minimum of one bottle per week to remind your baby how to take the bottle, but give as many bottles as you'd like. Substituting bottle feedings for breastfeeding allows Mom to sleep through the night and leave the house when she wants to.

What if you want to introduce a bottle before your baby is two weeks old? If your milk is in and your child is latching on, you won't have a problem going back and forth between the breast and the bottle. On the other hand, if you're not producing enough milk for your infant and you then offer a bottle, it may be difficult to get her back on the breast.

Common Sense Bottom Line

Try to wait until your infant is two weeks old before introducing a bottle; but if you can't wait that long, it's not the end of the world. If your baby is doing well with breastfeeding, she'll still take the breast even if she's had bottles. Remember, it's not nipple confusion, it's nipple common sense.

What If My Baby Refuses the Bottle?

It's best to offer at least one bottle a week beginning in the first month or so of your baby's life so that she gets used to it. Why do I suggest this? Because if she's totally breast-reliant, you may be in for a tug-of-war later on. A common scenario: Mom goes out for the evening. Dad tries to give the baby her bottle. The baby stubbornly refuses it. She's used to the breast whenever she wants it—and she wants it now. This isn't a mechanical problem; the baby knows how to suck from a bottle. It's an emotional issue, and it can become a battle of wills.

It makes sense that babies learn what their parents teach them, even if the lesson is unintended. If the baby learns that she'll be given Mom's breast whenever she refuses the bottle, it's not surprising that she'll hold out for the good stuff. This is often the case when moms return to work after a maternity leave. It is not uncommon to hear that the baby boycotted the bottle all day until Mom got home to breastfeed.

The only way to solve this problem is to stick to your guns. This is one behavioral lesson that if you teach it once, you won't have to teach it again. Here's what I recommend: Mom waits until right before a feeding (when the baby is most hungry), apologizes to whomever she is leaving the child with (because the baby is going to cry), then leaves the house and doesn't come back until baby takes that bottle. This may take an hour or, in the case of my daughter, eight hours. But I promise you: your baby will not starve herself. When she gets hungry enough, she'll take that bottle. After all the tears and trauma, she will have learned that when Mom isn't there, she's gotta drink from a bottle.

93

Daddy vs. Doctor—Refusing the Bottle

My daughter, Aubrey, had no problem going back and forth between breastfeeding and taking a bottle, either from me or my wife. But the day my wife went back to work, Aubrey—who was then four months old—refused to take the bottle from our babysitter. My wife called several times that day to check in, only to find that our daughter was on a bottle strike and alternating between fits of crying and sleeping. My wife was already anxious about her first day away from Aubrey, and now she was regretting returning to work altogether. Several times that day, she considered quitting her job. When she finally got home, Aubrey had gone eight hours without eating. My wife, who had also spent the whole day crying, hugged Aubrey and placed her on the breast to feed, which she did happily and voraciously. Unfortunately, all that my daughter learned that day was that if she held out for eight hours, the breast would finally appear. So it was no surprise that the following day Aubrey refused the bottle again. This time, after much debate, we waited to give her the breast until Aubrey finally took the bottle. We won, but it was a shallow victory. My wife and I hated to see our daughter crying and hungry. But after that second traumatic day, Aubrey had no problem taking the bottle from whoever offered it.

Should I Avoid Buying Baby Bottles That Contain BPA?

I have received a lot of questions recently about BPA, or bisphenol A, a chemical used to harden plastic, keep bacteria from contaminating foods, and prevent cans from rusting. Since BPA is used in bottles, sippy cups, and pacifiers, there is a fear that ingesting even small amounts could be harmful to an infant's development and reproductive function.

Many health and consumer organizations, including the FDA, feel that the amount of BPA ingested by infants and children is below that which would cause any harm. However, because of public outcry and a possible risk, further investigations are under way. Canada announced a ban on BPA in its baby bottles, and a number of major manufacturers in the United States, including Gerber and Playtex, agreed to stop using the chemical. The U.S. government is currently proposing a BPA-Free Kids Act.

I feel that there is probably too small an amount of BPA released to cause a problem, especially if you hand wash them and do not heat the container, but more studies need to be done. Since there are non-BPA options, if you are concerned you can forgo the risk. So how can you reduce your child's BPA exposure?

- Use baby bottles that are BPA-free plastic (usually opaque plastic)
- Avoid plastic containers that contain BPA
- Use glass bottles instead of plastic, but beware of the risk of injury from a broken bottle
- Don't microwave BPA-containing plastic bottles

Daddy vs. Doctor—BPA Bottles

After our daughter was born, we received several BornFree bottles (BPA free) as gifts. To be quite honest, we hadn't bothered to buy the BPA-free bottles because they were twice as expensive, and I didn't think it mattered. I figured that there was no scientific evidence that BPA causes problems in babies and that there is too small an amount of the chemical to be significant. I suspected that these new BPA-free bottle companies were simply preying on our fears.

Then I realized that my wife and I tended to give Aubrey mainly the BornFree bottles. My wife also expressed concern about heating the other bottles or putting Aubrey's plastic bowls or plates in the microwave. It made me think. My wife is not an alarmist, but she felt that an ounce of prevention was worth a pound of cure. I agreed. It couldn't hurt to offer only BPA-free containers to our daughter.

> Did we throw out everything else? No. I just wash them by hand and try not to heat them. I tell my patients, "If you have been using the BPA-containing bottles, don't worry. Your child will be fine. But it doesn't hurt to minimize your baby's exposure as much as possible." We do.

Help! Which Nipple Should I Buy?

The range of choices for bottle nipples is more extensive and confounding than a Starbucks menu. In addition to low flow, high flow, and small, medium, and large, nipples come in a myriad of shapes, colors, and sizes. Not to mention that some are orthodontic approved. One nipple has even been molded to look and feel like a real breast.

There's no need to spend a lot of money on different nipples. I know of families that spent hundreds of dollars trying different nipples only to find that the one they received free from the hospital works the best. When you do buy a nipple, start with a level one, which mimics the flow of the breast and minimizes your child's risk of choking or gagging. As your child gets older and stronger, gradually introduce a faster-flow nipple. There is no specific age or weight at which this transition should be made. Just pay attention to whether your baby seems frustrated by the slow flow and wants to drink faster. If this is the case, she may be ready for a faster-flow nipple. Just make sure that the milk isn't going into her mouth so quickly that she chokes or gags. No matter how fast the flow, be conscientious about pacing and monitoring your infant during feeding.

Common Sense Bottom Line

Don't worry about the type of nipple, but pace the flow.

The Ins and Outs of Breast Pumping

How Should I Deal with the Ordeal of Breast Pumping?

When to pump and how much to pump—these are only a couple of the concerns you may have about this modern-day wonder: the breast pump. But it doesn't have to be an ordeal. So let's tackle your concerns one at a time.

- *When should I pump?* It may seem counterintuitive, but the best time to pump is immediately after breastfeeding. That's because no infant empties the breast fully, and by pumping after the feeding you are emptying the well, so to speak, and sending a signal to your brain to produce more milk. The more you pump, the more milk you will produce (see below for how to deal with engorgement if you have more milk than you need). This is ideal if you are planning to store breast milk for future bottle feedings. You can begin pumping, for this purpose, as soon as your milk comes in. However, since you are going to start offering bottles when your infant is two weeks old, you may want to consider spending those first two weeks firmly establishing breastfeeding without the added time and stress of pumping.
- *How often should I pump?* The rule of thumb is to pump as much as you want to store in bottles. Some days you may want to pump after every feeding, other days not at all.
- *What time of day should I pump?* I recommend pumping mainly during the day. Nighttime is your chance to get a little sleep and recuperate. If you pump after every feeding around the clock you may find yourself exhausted, sleep deprived, stressed, and hungry. To ensure an optimal milk supply, it's very important that you eat and drink properly and get enough sleep.
- *Can I pump to relieve engorgement?* Yes, but not fully. For instance, let's say your baby starts to sleep longer stretches through the night (how wonderful!), but you wake up

97

engorged and in pain because your body thinks you are supposed to be breastfeeding. Pump out just enough milk to relieve your engorgement and pain, rather than the full amount your baby used to take during the night. This will tell your body to slow down your production of milk. And don't worry, just because you slow down production at one point doesn't mean you won't have enough when you need it. You will. Your body responds to your breast's stimulation so that you'll have the amount of milk you need for your child.

Common Sense Bottom Line
Pump immediately after breastfeeding. Pump mainly during the day. Pump as much as you need to store in bottles. Pump just enough to relieve the pain of engorgement, but not fully.

What If I'm Not Producing Enough Milk?

Some moms don't produce enough breast milk to satisfy their babies' needs or find that their milk supply diminishes at certain times, especially at night. If you are faced with either problem, make sure you are taking good care of yourself by following these guidelines:

- *Stay hydrated.* If you aren't drinking enough, your body can't produce enough milk. So drink, drink, drink.
- *Decrease your stress level.* Stress hormones inhibit milk production, so whatever you need to do to de-stress, do it. Get out of the house. Visit with friends. Exercise or do yoga.
- *Get some sleep.* Sleep allows your body to rejuvenate and is essential for a good milk supply.
- *Try home remedies.* Although not medically proven, these may help and are worth a shot. Mother's Milk Tea and fenugreek tabs can be found at your local drugstore or grocery store. Oatmeal is even considered to be helpful by many.

Once you've begun taking care of yourself, start pumping. Pumping your breast milk is probably the best way to increase your milk supply. Remember to pump as soon after breastfeeding as possible. You may find that you don't get much milk initially, but after a while your milk supply should increase. You may even consider consulting with a lactation specialist at your local hospital or lactation center.

If none of the above works . . . don't be afraid to supplement your milk with formula. Breast or bottle, breast milk or formula, your baby is going to be fine.

Now That I Have Enough Milk, How Long Can I Store It?

The advice you receive on how long you can store breast milk can vary greatly. Keep it simple and follow the rule of 5s. Breast milk may sit out on the counter for 5 hours, be kept in the refrigerator for 5 days, or stored in the freezer for 5 months. If you are not sure if the milk is good, smell it. If it does not smell right, discard it. It is not uncommon for the milk to adopt the smell of the plastic freezer bag.

Common Sense Bottom Line

Take steps to take care of yourself . . . and start pumping. It's the best way to increase your milk supply. And if all else fails, don't worry! Just supplement your milk with formula.

When to Stop Breastfeeding

How Much Longer Should I Breastfeed?

Unfortunately, moms often feel guilty about stopping breastfeeding "too soon." But when is too soon? Does the infant who breastfeeds for three weeks receive the same benefits as the one who breastfeeds for six months? Will you create a supergenius who never gets sick if you breastfeed longer?

Because of the many well-established benefits of breastfeeding, the American Academy of Pediatrics currently recommends exclusive breastfeeding for approximately the first six months of life and continued breastfeeding for the first year and beyond as

99

long as mutually desired by mother and child. That being said, it doesn't mean that an infant who breastfeeds for six months is guaranteed admission to a more prestigious college than the one who breastfeeds for only three. Or that the child who breastfeeds for nine months will have fewer infections than the one who does not breastfeed at all. It is merely that the longer you breastfeed the greater chance your child has to reap the benefits of breast milk. I agree that we should encourage mothers to breastfeed for as long as possible, but we should not make parents feel bad if they choose not to do so.

My feeling is that whether you decide to breastfeed one day, one month, or one year, you should feel comfortable with your decision. Yes, I believe breast milk is best for your baby. But I also feel that mothers already put too much pressure on themselves to do what's absolutely best for their children; they don't need more rigid guidelines. With the added benefits of omega-3 fatty acids such as DHA, formulas are better then ever—giving formula will not do your child a disservice. So breastfeed as long as you can, and if you need to stop because you are going back to work or it's uncomfortable or too much work or you're not producing enough milk for your child or whatever your reason, then stop. And don't feel guilty about it.

Common Sense Bottom Line

Breastfeed as long as you can, don't feel guilty when you stop, and don't let anyone make you feel guilty about your decision. Do what works best for you and your family. Your infant will be fine either way.

Daddy vs. Doctor—Two Hands Are Enough

Prior to Aubrey's birth my wife was resigned to the fact that she was not going to breastfeed. After all, her mom breastfed her for only two weeks and she turned out great.

As a pediatrician, this was hard for me to swallow, and part of me hoped she might eventually change her mind. During my wife's pregnancy, several of her friends had children and raved about their experiences with breast-feeding, so my wife decided she wanted to try. Shortly after birth, Aubrey latched on to the breast without a problem. Everything was going well for the first two weeks. She was eating, sleeping, and pooping without incident. Then one day at work I received a frantic phone call from my wife. She was in tears. I asked if everything was okay and she quickly responded, "No. Your mom and my mom have their hands on my breast and I have no room for my hands or Aubrey's head. I know they are trying to be helpful but this is stressing me out." That night Aubrey woke up for her usual two a.m. feeding but instead of going right back to sleep she was hysterical. My wife noticed that she was not producing as much milk as normal and we did not have any stored breast milk. She tried pumping, but the well was dry. My daughter was crying and hungry, and my wife was stressed and in tears. At three a.m. I got in the car and drove to the drugstore to pick up some formula. Neither of us wanted to do it, but it was what we needed to do at that time. Once my wife's stress decreased, her milk returned and she was able to successfully breastfeed Aubrey again. We realized that sometimes you have to do what is in the best interest of your child even if it deviates from your initial plan.

Introducing Formula

Is It Okay to Switch Between Breast Milk and Formula?

Of course. And yet, I have seen mothers brought to tears at the thought of having to give anything other than breast milk to their child. It's a shame, because feeding your baby formula is perfectly okay. If you can't breastfeed at every feeding time, your child will still thrive. And who says it has to be all or nothing? You might want to breastfeed during the day and give a bottle of formula at night so Dad can become part of the routine. Sometimes, when mothers go back to work and don't want to go through the hassle of pumping or don't have the time to, they may breastfeed in the morning and at night, and have the caretaker give bottles of formula during the day. Other families tell me that they give a bottle of formula at night to help their child sleep an hour or two longer. Since breast milk empties from a baby's stomach more quickly, breastfed infants get hungry more often, usually about every two to three hours, while formula-fed babies may make it three to four hours between feedings.

Common Sense Bottom Line
If you want to switch off between breast milk and formula, go ahead. Your baby will be fine.

Are All Formulas Created Equal?
There are some similarities between formulas and some major differences. All formulas for full-term infants have the same number of calories as breast milk. However, the type of protein, sugar, and additives may differ greatly. There are cow's milk protein formulas, soy formulas, hypoallergenic formulas, and formulas that are lactose-free. Some formulas claim to reduce gas and vomiting or mimic breast milk more precisely. Each formula manufacturer wants you to believe that its product is the "best tasting" and "most satisfying"—claims that begin to sound like beer commercials. All the hype can be very confusing. So let's cut through the adspeak and clarify why and when to use different types of formulas.

One of the main differences between breast milk and formula is the protein component. Breast milk is composed of a human milk protein whereas formula is composed of cow's milk protein.

Formulas with Cow's Milk Protein

- Similac Advance
- Enfamil Lipil
- Good Start Supreme
- Horizon Organic
- Kirkland brand

Don't be fooled by the brand names; they are all cow's milk protein formulas.

Some parents draw the false conclusion that if the formula doesn't agree with their infant, she must be lactose intolerant. In fact, when an infant is allergic to a formula she is usually allergic to the cow's milk protein in it. This has nothing to do with lactose, which is the sugar component of dairy products and formulas.

Signs of a Cow's Milk Protein Allergy

- fussiness with feeding
- taking a couple of sips and pulling away, then trying it again because the baby is hungry
- an increase in gas or fussiness during or immediately after feedings
- writhing and crying during and after feeding
- resistance to taking the bottle
- feeding well from the bottle with breast milk, but extremely fussy and pained with formula

More Severe Signs of a Cow's Milk Protein Allergy

- hives
- bloody stool
- weight loss or failure to gain weight

If a Cow's Milk Protein Allergy Is Suspected

- Do not simply change to a different cow's milk protein brand.
- Change to a soy formula or a hypoallergenic formula, depending on the severity of your baby's symptoms.
- If your baby's symptoms are not severe, switch her to a formula with a soy protein. Some examples of soy formulas include:

  - Prosobee (Enfamil's brand)
  - Isomil (Similac's brand)
  - Good Start Soy

- Cow's milk protein and soy protein are very similar, and 10 to 15 percent of infants who are allergic to cow's milk protein are also allergic to soy protein. If your infant still has symptoms of an allergy with the soy formula, switch to a hypoallergenic formula.
- If your baby's symptoms are severe, such as blood in the stool or failure to thrive, don't try the soy formula. Instead, skip right to a hypoallergenic one. Hypoallergenic formulas break up the cow's milk protein into smaller pieces so that the body can more easily digest them. Hypoallergenic formulas include:

  - Nutramigen (Enfamil's brand)
  - Alimentum (Similac's brand)

- Be aware that the hypoallergenic formulas are much more expensive and don't smell or taste very good. If your baby is still having problems on a hypoallergenic formula, she should be seen by a pediatric gastroenterologist for further evaluation. She may need to be started on an even more refined formula.
- When trying out a new formula, let your baby stay on it for at least three to four days to make sure that the previous protein has been totally eliminated from her system.

Milk Allergy Diagnosis and Treatment

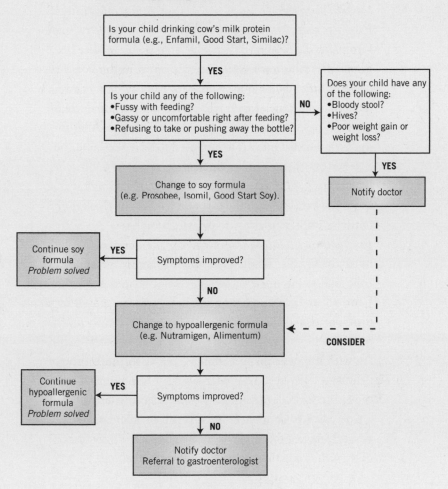

Is your child drinking cow's milk protein formula (e.g., Enfamil, Good Start, Similac)?

YES

Is your child any of the following:
• Fussy with feeding?
• Gassy or uncomfortable right after feeding?
• Refusing to take or pushing away the bottle?

NO → Does your child have any of the following:
• Bloody stool?
• Hives?
• Poor weight gain or weight loss?

YES

YES → Change to soy formula (e.g. Prosobee, Isomil, Good Start Soy).

Notify doctor

Symptoms improved? — **YES** → Continue soy formula *Problem solved*

NO

Change to hypoallergenic formula (e.g. Nutramigen, Alimentum) ← **CONSIDER**

Symptoms improved? — **YES** → Continue hypoallergenic formula *Problem solved*

NO

Notify doctor Referral to gastroenterologist

Now that you know when to use regular, soy, and hypoallergenic formulas, you should also be aware of other formulas you'll come across at your local market.

- *Lactose-free formulas:* Lactose is the sugar that is contained in all dairy products. The main reason to use a lactose-free formula is when your baby has a diarrheal illness, since dairy products exacerbate diarrhea. Once her stools are normal again, you can switch back to her normal formula. (You could also switch to a soy formula

105

when she's ill with diarrhea, since soy formulas do not contain lactose.)

- *Formulas that claim to decrease reflux or vomiting:* One such formula is Enfamil AR. The AR stands for "added rice." Some of our moms used to put rice cereal in the bottle to decrease spit-up or reflux. Similarly, Enfamil AR is a formula that thickens when it reaches the stomach to decrease reflux. It has the same number of calories as the other formulas and breast milk. It is supposed to have the same consistency of other formulas, thickening only when it reaches the stomach. Unfortunately, some parents report that this is not the case and that the formula tends to be thick in the bottle as well. So make sure you stir it well.

- *Formulas that claim to be a remedy for gas and colic:* No formula treats colic because we do not know the cause of colic, and as far as we know, colic is not related to feeding. Some formulas may treat an infant's gas if it's caused by a formula-related allergy. One such formula currently on the market is Gentlease, which is only partially hypoallergenic. As with hypoallergenic formulas, the cow's milk protein is broken down and washed, making it less allergenic, but the entire formula is not broken down. So if your baby has a true cow's milk allergy she will still be allergic to Gentlease. I suggest this formula for babies with mildly fussy or gassy symptoms that don't occur at every feeding.

Common Sense Bottom Line
Start with cow's milk protein formulas. Switch to a soy or hypoallergenic formula depending on your baby's symptoms. Switching brands is not the answer.

Why Are Omega-3 Fatty Acids So Beneficial for My Baby?

You may have noticed that omega-3 fatty acids are being added to almost everything these days, including baby formula. In fact, all the formulas now include it—they're the "Lipil" in Enfamil Lipil, the "advance" in Similac Advance, and the "supreme" in Good Start Supreme. Omega-3 fatty acids are important because of docosahexanoic acid (DHA), a fatty acid that is an important component of the growing brain. Numerous studies have shown improved visual and cognitive outcomes with DHA supplementation, as well as improved gross and fine motor skills, and improved weight and height gain in premature infants. Omega-3 fatty acids also support immune system development and function. Emerging data support a link between omega-3 fatty acids and respiratory health.

It is important to begin supplementation with DHA in pregnancy, because the brain grows 260 percent in the third trimester. But it's also important to make sure that infants receive it once they're born, because the brain grows another 175 percent in the first year of life, then 18 percent in the second year, and only 21 percent thereafter. Since synthesis of DHA in our body is extremely low (less than 1 percent), we must look to our diet for supplementation. Infants receive omega-3 fatty acids either through breast milk or formula with added DHA. As you would expect, the greater your intake of DHA, the higher the concentration found in your breast milk. Dietary sources of DHA include fish, eggs, and myriad foods to which DHA has been added, from pasta to baby food, and DHA supplements.

Common Sense Bottom Line
The more DHA the better. If you're breastfeeding, make sure you include it in your diet and/or supplements. If you're using formula, they all include it to varying degrees (check the label).

Can I Give Her Water or Juice?

Many parents are concerned that their infant may need supplemental hydration when it is hot outside. They frequently report that their own parents are pushing them to give the baby a little water. However, during the first six months of life, water is unnecessary even if you live in a hot climate or it's summertime. Do not worry. Your infant will stay adequately hydrated with breast milk or formula, and if she is thirsty she will just drink more of it. Introduction of water in a sippy cup with solid foods after six months of age is okay and will be discussed later in the chapter. No child needs juice in the first year of life, if at all. Juice is loaded with sugar, which is not nutritious and can be detrimental to her teeth. Stick with breast milk or formula to satisfy her thirst.

Does She Need a Multivitamin?

Breast milk is a wonderful source of many vitamins and minerals; however, it is a poor source of vitamin D. As a result, vitamin D supplementation is recommended for all breastfed infants through the first year of life. Although vitamin D is also synthesized from sun exposure, most infants do not spend enough time in direct sunlight or wear sunscreen, both of which prevent vitamin D synthesis. Infants drinking approximately 32 ounces per day of formula receive adequate levels of vitamin D, which is well known for helping the body build strong bones, but also plays a key role in helping to prevent infections, cancer, and autoimmune disorders such as diabetes. One milliliter (1 dropper) of Poly-Vi-Sol contains the recommended daily allowance of 400 IU of vitamin D and can be purchased over the counter. One daddy note: Poly-Vi-Sol contains the B complex vitamins, which are notoriously foul tasting. If your child does not like the Poly-Vi-Sol, you can buy the better-tasting Tri-Vi-Sol, which contains the same amount of vitamin D but not the B complex vitamins.

Introducing Solid Food

When Can I Get Something Solid to Eat?

If you asked twenty different people, you'd likely get twenty different answers about how and when to introduce solid foods to your baby. There have been books dedicated solely to how, when, and in what order you should introduce solid foods. As you approach this stage in your child's development, you'll probably receive handouts from health care professionals and advice from relatives, play groups, and Mommy and Me classes outlining the exact ways in which you should approach introducing solids, as if it were a tight-rope act and one wrong step would be disastrous.

Here's the deal: there is no one right way. When it comes to introducing solid food to your baby, I have two rules:

1. Have fun, and
2. Worry about quality and let your child worry about quantity.

When you start introducing solid foods, it tends to be more of a learning experience for your baby than a nutritional one. You may be excited about offering her pureed veggies, but she'll be more fascinated by the challenge of grabbing the spoon out of your hand. Or she may reach for your fork with enthusiasm when you're eating but turn her head away when you offer her food. All of this is perfectly normal. Even if she seems finicky or refuses meals altogether, remember that this is a new process for her and she'll eventually discover the foods she likes.

On the other hand, you may have a child who chows down like a linebacker. Nothing to worry about here, either. If she loves to eat, great. If she doesn't, no problem. Just have fun with the process. Introduce a variety of nutritious foods and let your baby experiment with what and how much to eat. You may find yourself worrying that she's not getting enough to eat, but rest assured: I have never heard of a healthy child who has starved herself.

As you begin this new stage in your baby's life, remember that you want to encourage healthy eating habits. So rather than offering her five things at once, choose a few foods that you want her to try, and stick with those during that particular meal. Today's dinner may be squash and carrots. Tomorrow it may be macaroni and cheese. But if you keep offering different choices at one time, she'll learn that she can keep refusing food until she gets exactly what she wants.

With that said, do give her foods you know she likes, but try new things as well. And just because she refused a food in the past doesn't mean you can't offer it again. It may take ten to twelve tries before she takes a liking to spinach or squash or turkey. The food she hated last week may be what she most craves tonight.

Routine is also important. Establish regular mealtimes and a   **109** meal place, preferably at the table where you and your family eat. Your child loves routines, and she'll be happier and healthier if she learns mealtime habits that help her fit in with the family. Along these lines: shut off the TV during meals and don't chase her around the room in order to give her one more spoonful of dinner. I hear parents tell me all the time, "He'll eat whatever I put in his mouth if I give it to him while he's playing or watching TV. At least he's eating, right?" Sure, a baby will eat in this catch-me-if-you-can fashion, but what kind of message will you be sending? Do you want him to grow up to be someone who can only eat if he's in front of the TV? And if he knows you'll chase him around with a forkful of food while he plays, why would he ever choose to sit down at the table? It's more important for babies to learn healthy eating habits than to get a certain amount of food in their mouths at every meal.

I never tell parents that their baby has to have a certain number of calories, because I know that a child will eat what she needs to eat. Some days she may eat a lot, other days nothing at all. Believe it or not, it all works out.

Common Sense Bottom Line

Introduce a variety of foods, but no more than a few at each meal. Don't worry about how much your baby is eating. She'll eat what she needs. Establish a mealtime and place—no running after her with a spoonful of pureed peas. Don't obsess—have fun!

When Is the Right Time to Introduce Solids?

I think one of the reasons parents are so eager to introduce solid foods is the hope that it will help their baby sleep through the night. But the truth is that once a baby reaches about four months of age, she should be able to sleep a ten- or twelve-hour stretch at night without eating—regardless of whether or not solids are in her diet. If she's still waking up and crying after that age, she wants your attention, not the leftover piece of chocolate cake.

Another myth about babies and solid food is that when you notice them eyeing your food, it means they're ready to eat it. Sorry, not true. Infants are mesmerized by everything they see around them, especially if their parents or older siblings are involved.

And then there's the belief that because your grandparents fed beef stew to your dad when he was only a month old, your own baby should follow in Dad's footsteps. After all, didn't they often know best how to raise kids in "the olden days"?

Trust me, there is no rush. Introducing solid foods is more work for you and an absolute mess. Your baby may not be as interested as you think, and it will not help her to sleep through the night. So when is the optimal time to start?

Most babies begin to be developmentally ready to eat solids between four and six months old. At this age, many infants have improved head and neck control as well as oral motor coordination. They are able to sit better with support and they lose their tongue thrust reflex. (Prior to four months of age, if you try to put something in your baby's mouth, she will usually thrust it out with her tongue.) Still, I recommend waiting until six months. Your child is going to grow exactly the same whether you give her solid food or not. Remember, when you start solids it tends to be more of a learning experience than a nutritional one, so the quantity she takes in is only a small portion of her total caloric intake. Also, some babies are still in the process of gaining the developmental skills needed to eat solid foods in a safe manner. So why risk their being disinterested or choking or gagging on their food when there's no nutritional benefit?

With that said, if you want to try solids sometime between four and six months, go ahead. Whether you start solids at four months, six months, or beyond, here are some simple guidelines. Choose what works best in your family . . . and have fun!

The Grandparent Way

We all know parents or grandparents who say, "I gave you a pork chop when you were four months old and you turned out just fine." For years, doctors rejected the early introduction of certain foods and advocated a conservative, stepwise approach. The idea behind this was to offer more allergenic foods (like fish, eggs, and peanut butter) later in life in order to avoid allergic reactions. Well, it turns out that the "grandparent way" of introducing foods is the right way—not offering a pork chop at four months of age due to the choking risk, but a more liberal approach to the introduction of new foods can be beneficial.

Recent studies show that the introduction of solid foods after six months of age, even foods considered highly allergenic, have no bearing on future allergies. In fact, one of the reasons we are seeing more children with food allergies may be because we did not sensitize them to a variety of foods early on. Doctors tell parents to introduce their infants to dogs and dirty surfaces to decrease their risk of allergy and illness later in life, but this philosophy hasn't been extended to peanut butter and other allergenic foods. However, studies over the past several years have challenged the protocol. One study, comparing the rate of peanut allergies among children in the United Kingdom and in Israel, showed that children in Israel who were introduced to peanuts earlier and ate them more frequently and in larger quantities had almost tenfold fewer peanut allergies. A similar study in the United Kingdom concluded that children who were introduced to peanuts earlier in life (around thirteen months of age) had a lower incidence of peanut allergy than those who waited until three years of age.

So it appears we had it backward. Unfortunately, parents still hear the same strict guidelines on how to introduce solid foods:

- You must introduce rice cereal first.
- You must introduce one food at a time and wait three days between foods to monitor for an allergic reaction.
- You must give egg yolks before egg whites.
- You should not introduce peanut butter until the age of three.
- You cannot give your child any dairy foods until they are one year of age.
- You cannot offer your child fish until they are at least eight to ten months old.

Try not to follow the old rules and instead follow what I like to call the grandparent way. Introducing a variety of foods early on sensitizes your child and may actually *decrease* their risk of allergies to these foods later on, as well as create a better and more adventurous eater (if you don't give a food until your child is three they probably won't like that food as much as one they have been given all along).

Solid Food Guidelines: Six to Eight Months

I recommend starting by offering one solid meal a day. It doesn't matter whether it's breakfast, lunch, or dinner—whatever suits your schedule. Offer the solid meal first, then follow it with the breast or bottle. This makes the most sense because if the milk is offered first, your baby will fill up and not want the solid food. I know the question that pops up is, "But isn't the milk more important?" Bottom line: it doesn't matter. Again, worry about quality and let your child worry about quantity. If your baby eats more solids, she may drink a little less milk. If she doesn't eat much, she may take more milk. It all evens out.

When your baby is having only one solid meal a day, the amount of milk she drinks won't change. When she's eating two to three solid meals a day, don't be surprised if she's only taking a half to two-thirds the amount of milk she used to take. It's not uncommon for infants to drink sixteen to twenty-four ounces a day with three solid meals when they used to drink twenty-eight to thirty-two ounces. The point is: don't worry about it. Your job is to offer your baby food and drink. She'll decide how much. When she decreases calories from one source, she'll supplement with another.

As your child starts to do well with one solid meal a day, add a new one. Follow your child's cues. She may not be interested in solids at all, so you may want to take it more slowly. On the other hand, I have families who come in for their six-month visit and report that their child loves solids and is already having three solid food meals a day.

Again, it won't hurt your child if she starts off with more than one meal a day, but it is not necessary, either. Remember, this is a learning process, and there is no rush. Your baby has the rest of her life to eat solid food!

What Foods Should I Introduce First?

Much of the advice parents are given in regard to the introduction of solid foods has changed in recent years. Parents were commonly told to start with rice cereal because it was thought to be a good source of iron, could be made to the proper consistency, and is relatively hypoallergenic. However, recent studies have shown that the absorption of iron from rice cereal is actually poor, so if you choose to skip over it, be my guest. I have only one rule when it comes to what food to introduce first: It should have a pureed consistency. Anything lumpy may be a choking hazard for an infant learning to eat solids. Delaying the introduction of foods does not decrease your child's risk of allergy (and may actually increase it), so feel free to offer a wide variety of foods early on. You are not limited to fruit, vegetables, and cereal. For example, if you want to blend eggs, fish, meat, cheese, yogurt, citrus, and peanut butter and feed it to your child, it is okay (though not very appetizing).

Many of the old ways of introducing foods are practical. For example, some of the easiest foods to puree tend to be fruit, vegetables, and cereals, so they still make for good first foods. But the point is to try not to worry about strict rules and guidelines and have fun. If you do offer rice cereal, oatmeal, or barley, mix the cereal with breast milk, formula, or even water (although it may not taste as good) and always feed it to your baby with a spoon. Putting cereal in the bottle passively provides calories and doesn't teach your baby about eating solids.

Your child will let you know how much she wants. She may take one spoonful or one jarful or nothing at all. Follow her cues. Start with a thinner consistency to make sure your baby can tolerate the added thickness of food and coordinate the spoon. If she chokes or gags (especially if she's younger than six months old), she may not be ready. Hold off and try again in a couple of days (or weeks if she's younger than six months).

Some families are concerned about cereal because some contain gluten, so they want to skip ahead to fruits and vegetables. Although some children are sensitive to gluten, most are not. One exception is if your child has been diagnosed with celiac disease, an inability to digest gluten.

114   Whether you introduce cereal or other foods like fruits and vegetables, you'll probably hear many different strategies on how to do this, including this mysterious piece of advice: introduce one color at a time (all the red foods first, then the green ones, then the blue ones . . .). I have no idea what the basis for this suggestion is, but in my opinion it's ridiculous. Others may tell you that you shouldn't introduce all the sweet fruits first or your baby will then refuse the vegetables. This makes sense, but you don't have to be so rigid. Most people like sweets, but we don't boycott everything else.

It may take your child several tries to decide what she likes. The order in which you introduce particular foods doesn't matter. And again, you don't have to be rigid with this routine. For example, you may try squash for three days, then bananas for two days, then peas for four days, or give them all in the same day. And keep in mind that it's okay to break the routine and improvise. But don't forget to reintroduce foods that she may not have liked intially. My daughter hated cereal. (Have you ever tasted the stuff? Yuck!) So we tried it once, then switched to sweet potato the next night, which she loved.

Are Certain Brands Better Than Others—and What About Organic?

Is there a big difference between Gerbers and Beech-Nut, store-bought and homemade, organic and nonorganic baby food? Not in my opinion. Organic foods have never been proven to be any healthier than nonorganic. So whatever makes you feel the most comfortable, go with it.

Why Is a Sippy Cup of Water a Good Thing?

I recommend offering a sippy cup of water when introducing solid foods to your baby because solids tend to be constipating, and water helps to keep the stools soft. Don't expect young children to be savvy with the sippy cup, or even to be able to hold it on their own, but it is nice for them to be introduced to one because that is what you'll be weaning them to when they're about a year old.

You may hear about mathematical formulas delineating the exact amount of water your baby is allowed to have. Don't worry about it. There's little chance she'll overdose on water, so give her as much as she wants. Most infants will take a sip or two, then be more interested in the cup. On the other hand, use common sense. If she's drinking so much water that she refuses her milk, take away the water.

Should I Worry About Food Allergies?

Although not common, your child may have an allergy to something she eats. Doctors used to recommend waiting a few days between introducing new foods in order to monitor for an allergic reaction. This is no longer considered necessary, because an allergic reaction may or may not occur in that time frame, and you wouldn't introduce foods this way forever. If your child has a reaction, you can start eliminating the most-likely culprits and figure it out that way. Thankfully, serious allergies are not very common. You may end up introducing one food at a time anyway, because if you open a jar or make a batch of pureed solids, you will probably end up using that for a couple of days before you start something new. But if you choose to give peaches at lunch and chicken and rice at dinner, go right ahead and try not to worry about allergies.

There are a number of signs of food allergy, including:

- diarrhea
- rash
- vomiting
- swelling
- breathing problems

By and large, however, symptoms that you think are an allergic reaction are usually not. It may just be a coincidence that she broke out in a heat rash the day you started her on bananas. And just because she spits up her cereal doesn't mean she's allergic to it. So if you notice what you think is a "reaction" to a particular food, but it doesn't seem to bother your baby, hold off on offering the food for about a week and try again. If she gets the same reaction, notify your doctor.

The three most concerning signs of a true allergy are swelling, breathing problems, and big blotchy hives. If you see these reactions in your baby, refrain from offering the suspected food, give her Children's Benadryl, and notify your pediatrician. If your child is having breathing problems, call 911. Fortunately, these three reactions are not common, especially with fruits, vegetables, and cereals.

Parents often ask if they should avoid giving their baby food that they are allergic to themselves. In general, unless you have a true anaphylactic reaction—a severe reaction that involves difficulty breathing—to a particular food, it is probably okay to try giving it to your child. If you have a family history of anaphylaxis, I would recommend avoiding the food and having your child tested by an allergist.

When you start solids make sure to have Children's Benadryl in the house in case of an allergic reaction (I have included a dosing sheet for your convenience in the reference section, see page 266).

Solid Food Guidelines: Eight to Ten Months

At this age your child will begin to develop a pincer grasp and she'll love to pick things up and put them in her mouth. This is the age when I recommend starting finger foods. Some parents worry that their toothless eight-month-old might choke on finger foods, and you are right to be concerned. Whether your child has a couple of teeth or none at all, she will not be able to chew her food well, so it is important to monitor its size and dissolvability.

You'll probably want to start with a pea-sized piece and gradually increase the size of the food as your baby's coordination improves. When we started Aubrey on finger foods, I called my wife "The Electron Microscope" because the pieces she offered were so small you could barely see them. Remember to use common sense and think about whether the food will dissolve, so that no matter what your child puts in her mouth, it will melt. Most babies love puffed cereal and Cheerios, which may be unsinkable but they're also dissolvable.

I call this the restaurant age, because your baby can go out to dinner with you and eat almost anything on your plate. If you want to go out for Chinese food, mash up a wonton for her—go crazy. If you're having mildly spicy Indian food and want to give her a taste, fine. She may prefer her food a bit more bland, but it's fine to let her start trying the tastes and spices you eat. The one spice I would not add more of to your child's food is salt. It may not hurt her now, but whatever she gets used to is what she'll want and expect. An overly salty diet is not healthy for any of us.

Most of the foods that you normally eat can be given to your baby in mashed-up form. Meat, such as ground beef and ground turkey, work well. You can also mash up a small piece of chicken with a fork and offer it to her. Steak would require pureeing (sacrilegious in my book, but be my guest). Of course, you can buy baby food that has pureed meat in it, although it doesn't seem as appetizing to me.

If you haven't already, this is the age at which you can give dairy foods, including cheese, yogurt, and cottage cheese. Most children love pasta dishes such as macaroni and cheese. When I recommend the introduction of dairy foods, some parents tell me that they had assumed babies shouldn't have dairy products until they're a year old. What they're actually referring to is the recommended age at which babies can switch to drinking regular milk. And this is because regular milk is a poor source of certain vitamins and minerals, including iron, whereas breast milk and formula are loaded with everything babies need. Your child can eat anything made with milk since it will comprise only a small percentage of her daily food intake, but hold off on introducing regular milk until she has reached her first birthday.

Your child may also like eggs and soy products. Some people wait on eggs until their baby is a year old. I introduce them earlier because there is no evidence that introducing these foods after four to six months determines whether your baby will be allergic to them and some of the vaccines your child will receive at one are egg-based, and it is good to know whether she is allergic to eggs prior to that. It used to be recommended to introduce the less allergenic egg yolk prior to the egg white. This is no longer the case. Tofu (and other soy products) is not only a great source of protein, but it's soft and can be sliced into dissolvable pieces. I am not worried about the hormones in soy, which you may have heard can cause early development of breasts in your son, or precocious puberty. Many people, including vegetarians and those who are allergic to dairy products, eat large quantities of soy protein from day one—and they do just fine. There is no conclusive evidence that dietary soy hormones will adversely affect your child's development, reproduction, or endocrine function. So I wouldn't worry about feeding your baby soy products. But, if you don't want to give them to your child, then don't.

When you start introducing finger foods, you don't have to introduce one food at a time. Just watch for any reactions. Also, only put the amount of food in front of her that you want her to put in her mouth at one time. For example, if you put twenty Cheerios on her tray, she'll fill both cheeks full of Cheerios before she knows what to do with them. So just give her a few at a time. I also recommend offering foods off your plate at each meal, placing them on your child's tray and noting what she likes.

And here's a bit of advice you might not want to hear: let her play with her food. This is all a new experience for your baby. She'll be interested in the different shapes and colors, smells and textures. This curiosity is a good thing. Let her explore what she's about to put in her mouth—even if it never reaches her mouth. This is also a time for honing her coordination skills. Don't be surprised, for example, if she eats the pureed bananas but pushes out the larger pieces because they're not as easy for her to swallow. She may also be unable to coordinate placing the food in her mouth.

What if she's totally disinterested in actually eating the food? She may just want to finger paint with it or throw it on the floor. The initial stages of solid food experimentation will create an absolute mess, but try to join in the fun (watching her, not engaging in a food fight). If nothing else, your dog will be the best fed on the block.

After you have offered your child some finger foods, spoon feed her some baby food. After a while when you offer her the spoonful of baby food, she'll push you away because she'll want you to put everything in front of her so she can pick it up herself.

And don't worry if your baby doesn't take to finger foods right away. She'll take the finger foods when she's ready, whether it's at eight months or ten or even a year. (Nobody goes to college on purees!) Just keep offering and follow her cues.

Solid Food Guidelines: Ten to Twelve Months

By ten months of age your child can eat almost everything that you eat. Liberalize the solid foods you are giving. Introduce fish (even shellfish) if you have not already. It is a good source of protein and

119

omega-3 fatty acids. I still recommend waiting until she's a year old to introduce honey. Certain foods such as citrus, strawberries, and tomatoes contain or release histamine, the chemical in our body that causes allergic symptoms, which is why many people wait before introducing them. I have to admit that we gave Aubrey strawberries and tomatoes before she was a year old and they caused a red rash around her mouth, but she loved them and the rash did not bother her. So it is okay to introduce them before a year, just look out for allergic symptoms.

Of course you should wait until your baby is at least three years old to introduce foods that commonly cause choking, such as nuts, popcorn, whole grapes, carrots, and hard candy. Honey is deferred until one year, not because of allergy but because honey can carry botulism, which in a child under a year old may cause a severe decrease in muscle tone and respiratory depression.

Some of these recommendations may change in the next couple of years as more studies correlating food exposure and allergies come to light.

Common Sense Bottom Line

Start solids around six months of age.

At six to eight months old: *Introduce a wide variety of pureed foods. Delaying solid foods beyond six months does not protect against the development of allergies. Follow her cues as to how much to give her. Worry about quality, not quantity. This is also a good time to introduce a sippy cup.*

At eight to ten months old: *Encourage finger foods and liberalize her diet. If you have not already done so, introduce meat, dairy, fish, and eggs.*

At ten to twelve months old: *At the end of this stage, your baby's diet should include nearly all table foods.*

Wait to introduce:

- *honey until one year of age*
- *nuts, popcorn, chewing gum, whole grapes, carrots, hard candy, or hot dogs until three years of age (risk of choking)*

Remember to let food fall on the floor . . . and make meals fun!

Daddy vs. Doctor—Pickles and Potato Chips

We started our daughter on solid food when she was six months old, but not before my wife protested, "Do we have to start her on food? Breastfeeding is so easy!"

Aubrey showed all the signs of being ready to go for the solid stuff. She was sitting without support, grabbing at our plates when we ate, and she always seemed to want to put everything in her mouth.

Still, she wasn't at all interested for the first couple of weeks when we tried introducing solids. She would just turn her head and make a face. (Mission not accomplished.) Then there was the matter of the mess. My wife and I are both Type A personalities (one of us more than the other, but I won't say who), so we'd feed Aubrey holding a spoon in one hand and a washcloth in the other, more focused on keeping things neat than enticing Aubrey to eat. It definitely took some time for us to let go and allow our daughter to do what babies do so well: make a mess.

When we started to introduce finger foods at eight months, we were confronted with the same initial response: Aubrey wasn't interested. We would place a couple of Cheerios on her tray and she'd play with them until they were either scattered across the kitchen floor or stuck to her sweaty palms. She would grab at my food when I was eating, but when I tried to stick a piece in her mouth that was not pureed, she'd turn her head and make a face like I was torturing her. My wife and I would joke that our daughter was happy to put anything in her mouth except food.

Then one day my wife was holding Aubrey and eating a sandwich. Aubrey reached over to her mom's plate, grabbed a pickle in one hand and a potato chip in the other, and went for it. She licked the pickle and then the potato chip, looked at my wife, and gave that expression that children give when they think they're getting away with something illegal. Then it was back to the pickle and the potato chip. She went back and forth sucking on the two foods voraciously, as if we hadn't fed her in days. (So much for the low-salt rule.)

After that, Aubrey was off to the races, picking up whatever food we put in front of her and refusing anything we tried to put in her mouth. Like most developmental milestones, it was nice to witness her progress, but I reminisce about the days when we had more control.

121

CHAPTER 5

SLEEP

Rock-a-Bye Baby: Sleep Habits and Sleep Training

· ·

E at, sleep, poop. These three mundane activities make up most of your baby's daily agenda. Of course there are all sorts of fun things she engages in as well, like making cute faces, throwing Cheerios on the floor, and constantly learning new stuff from Mom and Dad. But none of this would be possible without sufficient sleep. And babies need lots of it. In fact, it's not unusual for infants to sleep twenty hours a day in the first few weeks. They also wake up every few hours during the night needing to be fed or held or changed, so most new parents tend to be sleep deprived in the first two to four months of their baby's life. Which brings us to the question posed desperately by exhausted moms and dads: "When will she be able to sleep through the night?"

In this chapter, I'll answer that burning question, and in the process fill you in on the most important first-year sleep issues, including:

- Establishing a bedtime routine
- Setting a nighttime sleep goal
- Teaching your baby to self-soothe
- Scheduling naptimes

I'll also provide a common sense sleep-training recommendation:

• The Five-Ten-Fifteen Technique

And, finally, I'll familiarize you with:

• Necessary steps to prevent sudden infant death syndrome (SIDS)

It's Time for Bed!—Establishing a Bedtime Routine

It is never too early to establish a bedtime routine, and you can begin to do this when your baby is as young as two weeks old. By then she will have established her own feeding schedule, usually every two to four hours, and will be sleeping for much of the time between those feedings. Your goal is to get her used to the idea of a distinct "bedtime"—separate from all her other sleep times. Our daughter loved the "three B" routine of bath, breast/bottle, then bed. So here's what you can do:

• *Designate the feeding that normally occurs between seven and nine p.m. as your baby's "bedtime."* This time of the evening is ideal because it will make it easy to transition into a similar bedtime when your child is older.

• *Make this feeding different from all the others.* Since feedings every two to four hours around the clock appear to be the same to your infant, it is important to make her bedtime feeding distinct in some way. For younger babies, you might give her a bath, play a lullaby CD (or sing one if you're so inclined), or turn on the musical mobile above her crib. For older babies, you can read a story and put on her pajamas after her bath. The idea is to define for you and your baby that bedtime is different from all other feedings and naptimes. This is nighttime . . . and time for bed.

123

● *Understand that repetition and routines are important.* Babies—and children of all ages—like routines. It makes them feel secure. As for the nighttime routine, it's important to lay her down when it is time for her to go to sleep, preferably in her own crib. This repeated regimen will help her understand that her crib is the place for sleep.

When Will She Be Ready to Sleep Through the Night?— Setting a Nighttime Sleep Goal

Your baby is ready to sleep through the night when she's about three to four months old—when she no longer needs to be fed around the clock. Once she arrives at this stage, her need for nighttime feedings is primarily one of comfort rather than hunger. In other words, she really doesn't need to wake up to feed every few hours, but she's in the habit of doing so. Changing her sleep habits to coincide with her maturing needs will depend on your response when she wakes during the night. More on that in a minute, but first let's set a nighttime sleep goal.

Once your baby is three or four months old, you can start to define her "nighttime period"—that is, what constitutes a healthy and reasonable night's sleep for a baby her age. Your goal is for her to get a minimum of ten hours of nighttime sleep (anything more is a bonus). If you have been putting her down at eight p.m., your baby's nighttime period would be defined as "eight p.m. to six a.m." (a ten-hour block).

Knowing that it's normal and healthy for a three- to four-month-old to get ten uninterrupted hours of sleep at night, and having set that goal for your baby, how can you help her to achieve it?

How Can I Teach Her Healthy Sleep Habits?—Teaching Your Baby to Self-Soothe

In the first three to four months of life, your baby learns that the world is a safe place. She learns this because when she's hungry, you feed her; when she has a dirty diaper, you change her; and when she cries, you pick her up. At around four months of age she enters a new phase of development, in which she discovers that she can do a little more on her own. This is the appropriate time for her to develop her independence by learning to soothe herself to sleep and to sleep through the night.

You can prepare your baby for this major learning step by beginning, when she's around three months old, to let her cry a little longer at night before you go in to pick her up. Decide on an amount of time you can listen to her cry without responding; it could be five minutes or even fifteen. Anytime she cries during the night, wait that amount of time to give her a chance to look around the room, realize that she's not hungry, and soothe herself to sleep. If she's still crying after the allotted time, go in and pick her up, feed her or comfort her. What usually happens between age three months to age four months is that she'll learn to go back to sleep on her own and skip some or all of the nighttime feedings. Waiting the five or ten or fifteen minutes until you go in to pick her up allows you to ease into the five-ten-fifteen technique.

At four months old, you're ready to go full force with your child's sleep training: no picking up and no feeding. If you've been easing her into the routine, your baby may be very close to sleeping through the night. If you haven't, or if she still isn't getting the hang of it, she will need your help to be an accomplished sleeper through the night.

How can you help her? The first important key is:

- Lay her down to sleep when she's still groggy, rather than when she is fast asleep.

Putting her down when she's partly awake allows your baby to learn that she can fall asleep on her own, without being rocked or bounced or needing a bottle or breast in her mouth.

There are entire books devoted to sleep training, but let's pare it down and make it simple. The key to teaching your baby to fall asleep on her own and to go back to sleep when she awakes during the night is to:

- Help her learn to soothe herself.

125

I know this may be easier said than done. Obviously, every parent would love for his baby to sleep through the night, but what about the myriad concerns that crop up, preventing well-intentioned moms and dads from following through with the self-soothing lesson? For instance:

Four (or six or eight or twelve . . .) months old is still so young!

My child eats voraciously throughout the night—I'll be starving her!

She doesn't weigh enough!

I'll be damaging her psychologically if I let her cry!

I don't want to give up the nighttime feeding—it's our special bonding time!

I understand your concerns; however, I assure you that it is absolutely safe to sleep train your child at four months old. If you don't want to, that's fine. It's possible that your baby will start sleeping through the night on her own . . . or maybe you won't mind being awakened by a two-year-old who continues to call out your name every few hours throughout the night or crawls into bed with you on a regular basis. But if you'd like your baby to learn how to soothe herself to sleep and to sleep comfortably on her own through the night, I'd like to recommend a technique that is based on Dr. Richard Ferber's sleep-training method. I refer to my version of this method as the Five-Ten-Fifteen Technique.

Common Sense Parenting Five-Ten-Fifteen Technique

In order for this technique to work, you need to commit to two basic rules:

1. You can't pick up or feed your child during the ten-hour sleep period that you've designated.
2. If you do check on her, you must extend your response time by five minutes each time you go into her room.

You may be rolling your eyes at this point, but bear with me. Here's how the five-ten-fifteen technique works:

1. Put your child to bed using the bedtime routine you've established.
2. The first time she cries during the ten-hour block of time you've designated, wait five minutes before you check on her. When you do check on her, touch her or talk to her and reassure yourself that she is not sick or hurt. If there is something to fix (like a wet diaper), fix it. Then, after no more than a few minutes, leave the room—even if your child is still crying, which she likely will be.
3. Understand that the reason she's still crying is that she didn't get what she has always gotten prior to your starting this technique: picked up or fed. She's not hungry and she's not in pain.
4. If she continues crying or starts crying later that night, wait ten minutes this time before checking on her. Then, as before, go in and touch her, talk to her, and leave within a few minutes.
5. If she continues to cry or starts to cry again later that night, wait fifteen minutes this time before checking on her. And go through the same touch, talk, and leave routine.

Remember, after the third time you go in to check on her, every time she cries or continues to cry after that, wait fifteen minutes until you check on her.

After the first night, up the ante and increase the intervals to ten-fifteen-twenty minutes. On the following night, increase them to fifteen-twenty-twenty-five minutes, and so on. You don't have to use these exact intervals, but the longer the interval you start with, the quicker your child will learn how to sleep through the night. If you choose not to respond at all when your child cries, she may learn to sleep through the night in one or two days. If you choose to respond more frequently, it will take her longer to adjust to soothing herself to sleep.

I realize that your first few nights of going through the five-ten- **127** fifteen technique won't be easy. Just remember that for the last four months your baby has always gotten exactly what she wanted, so give her time to adjust to the fact that your response has changed. She's used to believing that if she cries loud enough and long enough, you'll give in. It may take her a few nights or longer to make that adjustment.

The idea here is to get your baby used to awakening, looking around the room on her own, realizing that she's okay, and putting herself back to sleep. If you stick to the plan, she'll get past the traumatic first night or two, and by the third night she may only wake up once for a short time and go back to sleep. Within a week she'll be getting ten to twelve hours of sleep every night. And your whole family will enjoy more restful nights. This technique may not suit every family. However, every baby develops better, and is in a better mood, when she has a good night's rest. You, too, will be happier and better prepared for your day.

One last bit of advice: since initially there will be a whole lot of crying going on, I recommend that you pick a weekend to begin the five-ten-fifteen sleep-training technique. That way you won't show up at work even more sleep deprived than usual.

Common Sense Bottom Line

A baby over the age of four months who continues to cry in the middle of the night in the hopes of being picked up or fed is a lot like someone who plays the slots in Vegas. If she's won once, she'll keep playing. If your baby cries for three nights straight while you're trying to sleep train her, and on the third night you can't take it anymore and give in, she wins—and everything you accomplished prior to that point goes out the window. So stick with the five-ten-fifteen program. The payoff will be peaceful, silent nights for the whole family.

Remember, training your baby to soothe herself and fall back to sleep on her own is safe and advisable after four months. Letting her cry does no psychological damage—it merely teaches her something new and valuable.

Daddy vs. Doctor—Sleep Training

Everyone always asks me if, as a father, I can take my own advice. "You'll see," they say. "When you're a dad it's totally different." The truth of that statement was driven home when we were training our daughter to sleep through the night.

It was easy for me to discuss sleep training with parents. I didn't have to hear their child crying or watch the tears roll down her rosy cheeks. But when it came to Aubrey, how would I manage to hear her screaming in the next room, knowing that if I just picked her up we could all go back to sleep and be fresh for work in the morning?

My wife had heard me talk about sleep training with patients so many times that she could recite the instructions by heart long before we had our own child. In fact, her friends would often call her for advice. Before she was pregnant with Aubrey, she went to visit a good friend who had yet to sleep train her eight-month-old. When my wife came home from the trip, she was in a serious state of sleep deprivation, having listened to the friend's baby cry all night long for a week. Exhausted and cranky, she asked me, "When we have a baby, what's the earliest we can sleep train?" I answered, "Three to four months," and jokingly added, "but I want it in writing that you'll agree to it, because it's harder than you think." My wife shot me a confident look and replied, "No problem."

Fast-forward a year and a half. Aubrey had just turned four months old, and although she had always been a good sleeper, she was waking up several times a night. My wife and I decided it was time to start the sleep training. That Friday night, Aubrey went to sleep at seven-thirty and woke up crying at ten. My wife sat up in bed and grabbed the video monitor. She stared at the monitor and watched Aubrey cry. Because the crying was being brought to us in

129

stereo, it seemed even louder. Tears started rolling down my wife's face. She looked at me, calmly lying in bed watching TV, then back at the monitor. She looked at me again and demanded to know why I wasn't upset. I told her, "Because we know she's not hungry or hurt or sick. She's just looking for comfort."

In reality, I was dying inside as well. I wanted to run to Aubrey and pick her up. I wanted to be her hero and save the day, but I tried to stick to my guns. My wife, on the other hand, told me I was insensitive. How could I just sit there and watch TV with my daughter crying miserably in the next room?

After a few more minutes, she got out of bed in a huff, muttered "I can't do this," and went and picked up Aubrey.

Sleep training was aborted for the night.

The next day we hardly spoke. I was the insensitive father who lets his daughter cry, and she was the hypocritical mother who could give her friends advice but couldn't follow through with it herself. I mentioned the trip she had taken a year and a half earlier, and she shot me a glance that needed no words.

The following night we declared a truce and decided to try again. The night started off well. Then around ten Aubrey started to cry. We both sat up in bed and stared at the monitor. I said, "Just watch the clock. It seems like forever, but hopefully she won't cry that long." Aubrey cried for seven minutes then fell asleep. Four hours later she did it again and fell asleep. We held strong.

After a few nights of sporadic crying, our daughter was sleeping through the night. Sometimes she would cry for a few minutes, once she even cried for an hour and a half, but we didn't relent. We stared at the baby monitor in mild agony, but we held to our commitment to let her make it through the night on her own.

Each morning, I would walk into Aubrey's room and she

would be lying there looking up at me with a big smile on her face. She wasn't holding a grudge, and I doubt she'll hold it against us twenty years from now.

Sleep training our daughter wasn't easy. My wife and I both wanted to go in and rescue her each time she awoke crying, but we also realized that part of that urge was for our own selfish reasons. We knew that picking her up would not only make her feel better in that moment, it would also allow us to get back to sleep. In reality, though, what was best for Aubrey was to learn to self-soothe and sleep through the night. Nobody feels good when they don't get a good night's rest. Learning to sleep all night meant Aubrey would be a happier, healthier baby.

The following weekend I caught my wife on the phone explaining to a friend how to sleep train her baby—and how easy it had been for us.

The Lowdown on Naps

Most babies take three naps a day until around six months of age and two naps until around fifteen to eighteen months. The goal is an hour per nap—anything beyond that is a bonus. If your child has learned to sleep through the night, naptimes may fall into place on their own. If not, it makes sense to choose the times of day when your child is tired and fussy as her naptimes. If you pick roughly the same times each day, it will create a routine your child can depend on.

So here's how the nap routine goes:

- Put her in her crib at your designated naptime for one hour.
- During that hour, she can sleep, play, or even cry, but she has to stay in her crib.
- You can check on her if you want to, but don't pick her up or feed her.

131

· When the hour is up and your child is awake and calling for you, regardless of whether she slept, take her out of her crib and go on with your day.

· If she sleeps beyond an hour, that's fine; let her sleep. But don't let her sleep much more than three hours during any naptime. Otherwise, she may not sleep as long at night.

After a few days of the naptime routine, your child will learn to go to sleep during these times, and maybe sleep even longer than an hour.

Common Sense Bottom Line

Once your child is sleeping through the night, naptimes should fall into place. If they don't, you can use the five-ten-fifteen technique. Remember, babies need their rest . . . and they love routines.

Back to Sleep—Preventing Sudden Infant Death Syndrome (SIDS)

Yes, we slept on our stomachs when we were babies and lived to talk about it. However, I also used to sled down a hill in the winter across a busy street, but I do not recommend doing that anymore. Since the "Back to Sleep" campaign began in the early 1990s, instructing us to put infants to sleep on their backs, the incidence of sudden infant death syndrome (SIDS) has decreased by more than 50 percent.

SIDS, or crib death, is defined as any unexplained sudden death of an infant less than one year of age. It remains the number one cause of infant death in the United States beyond the neonatal period. SIDS peaks between two to four months of age and drops off precipitously after six months, with 90 percent of SIDS deaths occurring before six months.

We don't know the exact cause of SIDS, but the prevailing belief is that certain infants have an immature brain stem that does not arouse them during pauses in breathing. If an infant has this pre-

132

disposition and is placed in her crib in a position that could lead to suffocation, such as on her stomach, this may cause sudden infant death. Most of us slept on our stomachs and were fine because we didn't have the brain stem predisposition. Since we don't know which infants are susceptible, it is important to put all children to sleep on their backs.

I know some parents worry about their babies spitting up or vomiting in their sleep and choking themselves, but this was investigated and found not to be a valid concern. Healthy infants will automatically swallow, cough, gag, or turn their head when they spit up. There has been no increase in choking deaths due to back sleeping.

There are a number of preventive measures that can reduce your child's risk of SIDS. If you follow these precautions, you'll have little to worry about.

- *Back to sleep:* The single most important precaution is to place your baby on her back when you put her down to sleep. Avoid side sleeping as well, which can lead to her accidentally rolling onto her stomach. Parents frequently express concern that when their child is old enough she can roll over on her own onto her stomach in the middle of the night. They wonder if they need to keep rolling her back onto her back. At this age, usually four months or older, her SIDS risk has decreased and she is strong enough to roll over and lift her head. I still recommend placing her to sleep on her back, but if she rolls over onto her stomach, she is safe to stay there. The only alternative would be to sleep next to her crib and reposition her all night long.
- *The firmer the better:* Always have your child sleep on a firm mattress or sleep surface and avoid soft pillows or loose blankets that may be suffocating.
- *Avoid the abominable snowman:* Although your baby looks cute bundled in her furry onesie like the abominable snowman, avoid overbundling her. Instead, dress her in light sleepwear. Her bedroom should be a comfortable temperature, and she should not feel hot to the touch.

133

• *Avoid bumpers:* Bumpers were invented to prevent infants from getting their arms and legs stuck between the bars of their cribs. Now that government regulations require cribs to have a safe bar width, bumpers don't serve any safety purpose. Yes, your child may bump or bruise her head against the bars, and yes, decorative crib bumpers are an aesthetic touch, but studies mention a possible risk to babies. The truth is, before four months old, infants can't roll over toward the bumpers so it's a moot point. After four months old, they can roll over, and the bumpers could cause suffocation. So if you really want those cute bumpers, use them only in the first few months. Remove them by the time your child is four months old. Also remove any stuffed animals or pillows, as they could cause suffocation as well once the baby can roll over.

• *No smoking:* Maternal smoking during pregnancy, as well as secondhand smoke after the baby is born, are risk factors for SIDS. Don't smoke!

• *Avoid co-sleeping:* You may love cuddling and being close to your infant while you sleep, but co-sleeping risks accidental suffocation because of rolling over on your baby or throwing a pillow or blanket over her. Instead, you can have her sleep in her crib next to your bed. Having your infant sleep next to your bed may actually decrease the risk of SIDS.

• *Avoid commercial devices:* Some companies claim to have devices that prevent SIDS or alarm you so that you can intervene prior to something bad happening. These electronic respiratory and cardiac monitors should be avoided for two reasons. One, they will keep you up all night worrying about false alarms. And two, they are not proven to be effective in reducing the risk of SIDS.

• *Consider pacifier use:* Sucking on a pacifier may keep your child in a more aroused state, thus decreasing her risk of SIDS. I don't recommend introducing a pacifier solely for this purpose, but if she is already using one, think of its SIDS-prevention capability as an added benefit.

134   • *Avoid excessive time in car seats or bouncers:* Car seats and

bouncers are often very cushy and place the body in a position with the head and neck flexed forward and the airway crimped, so it's best to avoid long periods of time in these devices.

* *Educate:* One-fifth of all SIDS deaths occur in the presence of a secondary caregiver, so make absolutely certain that nannies, day care attendants, and babysitters are aware of the risk factors for SIDS—and that they know to place baby on her back when she goes down for a nap.

Common Sense Bottom Line
Follow the above preventive measures to lower the risk of SIDS.

Daddy vs. Doctor—Back to Sleep

When Aubrey was four and a half months old, we would put her to sleep on her back, and as we were walking out of the room she would roll onto her stomach. If we flipped her back over, she would wake up, cry, and roll back over onto her stomach again. For several nights after her first rollover, I went in to check that she was still breathing, and my wife would turn on the video monitor sound to the highest setting to make sure she could hear Aubrey. (I got used to sleeping through the sound of static.) As a doctor I knew that by the time a baby can roll over, there is less need to worry about SIDS, because the child is neurologically and developmentally more advanced. We continued to put her to sleep on her back but knew whatever position she found herself in was one in which she was safe.

CHAPTER 6

POOP

The Scoop on Poop

· ·

Oh, poop. I have answered so many questions about poop that sometimes I feel I'm standing waist-deep in it. For some reason, this simple biological function scares parents to death. It's hard to figure out why parents are so concerned with their baby's poop that they feel compelled to agonize over it, scrutinize it, smell it, and in some cases even taste it!

I remember one night I received an emergency page from an anxious father who reported that his six-month-old's poop *tasted* different. I assumed I had misheard him, so I asked him to repeat what he'd just said. He answered, "My son's poop tastes different."

This had to be a joke. *Different from what?* I thought. Then I asked him, "Why did you taste your son's poop?"

He answered, "Because it smelled different."

I continued with a few more questions and came to the conclusion that this man's son was just fine. My suggestion: that Dad stop examining his son's bowel movements so closely—and definitely stop tasting them.

Everything you need to know about your baby's poop can be covered fairly easily, which is what I plan to do in this short chapter. We'll go over:

- What is poop?
- Why does poop look and smell different at different times?

- What is the normal frequency of a baby's bowel movements?
- Why do babies get constipated—and what you should do about it?
- Why do babies get diarrhea—and what you should do about it?

I'll also offer you my Common Sense Doo Doo Doctrine so that you'll know what to be concerned about and what is perfectly normal.

What Is Poop?—Poop Defined

Poop is what is left over after you eat and your body has absorbed the nutrients from foods that it needs. And just like the trash sitting in your garbage can, poop may be many different shapes, sizes, colors, smells, and even consistencies.

An infant's poop starts off as a tarry black material called *meconium,* which is all the stuff your child swallows when she is in her mother's womb. As the infant begins to feed, the milk is digested and the meconium is pushed out of her body. At this point, her poop is a transitional green color; then it changes to a mustard yellow. These changes usually correspond with the breast milk supply increasing, when your baby is around three to five days old. The mustard yellow poop may be very watery at first and occur after every feeding, especially in breastfed babies. As your child gets older, her poop may change color, consistency, smell, and frequency depending on her diet, her mother's diet, and her own digestive system.

If you follow the Doo Doo Doctrine, you'll know which poop issues require a phone call to your doctor.

Doo Doo Doctrine

The color, smell, consistency, and frequency of poop should not alarm you, unless you see one of the following signs—in which case, you should contact your pediatrician:

- **_The poop is black and tarry after the meconium has already changed to normal poop._** This may be a sign of digested blood in the stool. It is normal to have very dark brown or army green stool, but not black and tarry.

- **_The poop has bright red blood in it._** This may be a sign of undigested blood in the stool.

- **_The poop is white._** This may be a sign of a rare liver disorder that is first noticed in the first few months of life.

- **_The poop is pure water and your child is not urinating._** This may be a sign of diarrhea. It is common for infants to have watery, seedy stools more than ten times per day. As long as your baby is drinking and staying hydrated, diarrhea is not a concern.

- **_The poop is hard as a rock._** This may be a sign of constipation. Remember, it is normal for a baby to grunt and strain when she poops, and this does not necessarily mean she is constipated. But if the stool comes out as hard rocks, notify your pediatrician.

What If My Baby Strains When She Poops?

All babies strain and turn bright red when they poop. This is because they do not know what muscles to use to push out the poop, so they strain in order to find the right ones. Although this straining may last several months, it is not necessarily a sign of constipation or pain. If the poop comes out soft, your baby is not constipated.

What About Frequency? How Often Is Often Enough?

Whether your child poops ten times a day or once a week, both patterns are normal.

At a baby's two-week visit, I often discuss poop and bowel patterns with new parents. When I tell them that their infant, who has been pooping ten to twelve times a day, may slow down to once or twice a day or even once or twice a week, I always get the same look of disbelief and alarm. I explain that such variations are perfectly normal. Breast-fed babies usually start off pooping more frequently in the first couple weeks of life and then slow down, while formula-fed babies tend to poop more frequently at that time. As long as she is not having hard painful stools it does not matter if she poops ten times a day or once a week. Everyone's gastrointestinal system works differently. As long as she is urinating then you know that she is staying hydrated—poop does not really matter. If it is not bothering her, do not let it bother you.

Common Sense Bottom Line

If your child poops ten times a day or once a week; has watery, seedy, Play-Doh or soft-serve ice cream consistency poop; has poop that smells like roses or rotten eggs; or has poop that is green or yellow or brown—it is all perfectly normal.

Daddy vs. Doctor—Where's the Poop?

My wife had heard me give the advice to new parents about a baby's changing bowel patterns so many times that I assumed when our own baby's habits started changing she'd know everything was as it should be. Boy, was I wrong.

Our daughter was a regular pooper for the first three months and then . . . she went two days without pooping. She was happy and playful, just no poop. My wife turned to me and asked, "Where's the poop?" It sounded like the old Wendy's commercial where the customer demands to know, "Where's the beef?"

Although I realized that my wife knew there was nothing seriously wrong with Aubrey, our lives became consumed with poop. From that point on, after every moan, giggle, grunt, or hiccup, my wife would ask her rhetorically, "You gotta poop? You gotta poopy?" Dinner conversation that night centered on . . . poop. "Do you think she will go tonight or tomorrow?" Every time we mentioned the word "poop," I put a quarter in a jar for Aubrey's college fund. I am proud to report that poop has laid the foundation for our daughter's future education, and she now has ten dollars and seventy-five cents.

After two days of no poop, we were giving Aubrey a bath when all of a sudden there was that sound. The sound where a wife looks at her husband and says, "That's disgusting—go in the other room." But this time I heard my wife exclaim, "Thar she blows!" My first thought was, first a Wendy's quote now *Moby-Dick*. Then we looked down at Aubrey grinning ear to ear. It was the blowout of all blowouts—and it was all perfectly normal.

Constipation

Infants who are constipated may strain and cry when they poop because it is hard to get the poop out, and when they are finally relieved there is only a small hard stool to show for it. Constipation may occur in a child who only poops every two to three days or one who poops once a week. Frequency isn't the determining factor. Consistency is. If the poop is hard and associated with pain and straining, the problem is constipation.

True constipation in the first two months of life is not common and should be brought to the attention of your doctor immediately. I say "true" constipation because infants will commonly grunt and moan, strain and turn red during pooping, or skip days between pooping, but they aren't necessarily constipated. If their poop is not hard, it's normal.

After two months of age, if your baby has bouts of hard stools, you can do the following:

1. Make sure she's drinking enough. If she's not getting enough fluids, her poops may get hard. You could give her an ounce

or two of prune or pear juice to get things moving. The exact amount doesn't really matter. You just don't want to give her so much that it's substituting for her milk.

2. If she's formula-fed, try switching formulas. Cow's milk protein tends to be constipating, and this is the type found in most formulas (for example, Enfamil, Similac, Good Start). Try switching to a more broken down formula such as a partially hydrolyzed (Gentlease) or fully hydrolyzed formula (Nutramigen or Alimentum). Your infant may be able to digest these formulas more easily and resolve the constipation.

3. If she has already started solid food, steer clear of binding foods such as pasta, cereals, bananas, rice, apples, and toast. Instead, increase the "P" fruits: pears, plums, peaches, prunes, and apricots (second letter—close enough). "P" fruits help you poop. Also: offer her more water, decrease dairy products, and give her an ounce or two of prune or pear juice each day until her poops become painless and regular.

4. If the above suggestions don't work, you can try medications such as Milk of Magnesia, which are safe in children under a year old.

5. As a last resort for the child who is screaming in pain, an over-the-counter suppository, such as a glycerin suppository, is safe to try to get quick relief until you can talk to your doctor.

Common Sense Bottom Line
If your baby is under two months old and her poop is hard, indicating "true" constipation, call your doctor. Otherwise, don't worry. If your baby is more than two months old, try the aforementioned treatment options to soften your child's stool.

Diarrhea

Diarrhea is defined as a sudden increase in watery stools. In infants, diarrhea is usually caused by a viral infection called *gastroenteritis*. Diarrhea may be present alone or with a combination

141

of symptoms that include vomiting, fever, and abdominal cramping. It may last one to two weeks and is usually most severe in the first twenty-four to forty-eight hours. As you probably already know from treating yourself, the most important treatment for diarrhea is "plenty of fluids."

You may notice that your child's diarrhea is foul-smelling or a different color than her normal poop. This is to be expected and does not mean the infection is more serious. Diarrhea is often green because viral illnesses cause an increase in the transit time of things going through the intestines; the faster things go through, the greener they are. You may also notice that your baby has more severe and foul-smelling gas. Again, this is normal. Pick the side of the family you want to blame it on, then realize it will soon pass.

If your child has diarrhea, make sure to avoid all dairy products. Breastfeeding is still okay, but all other milk products are a no-no. Why? Because dairy products contain the sugar lactose, and when you have a viral gastroenteritis, the lining of the intestine, which is responsible for absorbing lactose, gets worn away. So if you give your child products that contain lactose they will go right through her and increase her diarrhea. If your child usually drinks formula containing lactose, switch her to either a lactose-free or soy formula. Both have the same nutrient values and number of calories as regular formula, but without the lactose. Continue these formulas until your baby goes three to four days without having diarrhea. If you reintroduce lactose before the intestines have had time to heal, you will exacerbate her condition.

If your child feels like eating solids, offer her a healthy, balanced diet. Physicians have moved away from recommending the BRAT diet (bananas, rice, applesauce, and toast) because we do not want to limit the diet of a child with an already limited appetite. Sure, starchier foods, such as pasta and rice, tend to be more binding, and bland foods, such as chicken soup, will be gentler on her stomach than spicy ones. Remember, it is absolutely normal if your child does not want to eat anything. So don't force her. She may lose weight, but she'll regain it when she's feeling better. The objective is to keep her hydrated with lots of fluids. You may also offer her a probiotic, such as acidophilus, which can be found over the counter. Avoiding restrictive diets by offering age-appropriate foods from a variety of sources, avoiding dairy, and supplementing with a probiotic will optimize your child's nutrition and maximize her recovery from a diarrheal illness.

And remember, not all loose stools are diarrhea. Breastfed infants often have frequent loose stools that may be indistinguishable from diarrhea. Still, you'll want to make sure that your baby is getting enough fluids so that no more is coming out than is going in. If she has frequent watery stools and is happy and drinking well with multiple wet diapers, it doesn't matter if we call it breastfed poop, runny poop, or full-on diarrhea. She's doing fine.

Common Sense Bottom Line
Remember hydration is the key, but steer clear of dairy products. Breastfeeding is fine. Don't be surprised if your baby does not want to eat and is drinking less than normal. Notify your doctor if your child has blood in her poop, fewer than three wet diapers in a twenty-four hour period, a fever for more than seventy-two hours, or is inconsolable.

Common Sense Facts: Diarrhea

What is diarrhea? Diarrhea is defined as a sudden increase in watery stool. It is usually caused by a virus and may last one to two weeks. Diarrhea may present alone or with a combination of symptoms that include vomiting, fever, and fussiness. The symptoms are usually most severe in the first twenty-four to forty-eight hours.

Breastfed infants
- Provide breast milk on demand, which may be more frequently than normal.

Formula-fed infants
- Avoid cow's milk–based formulas that have lactose (Enfamil Lipil, Simalac Advance, Good Start Supreme) until normal stools resume.

143

- Soy-based (Prosobee, Isomil, Good Start Soy) or lactose-free formulas are okay.
- If she is refusing her normal liquids, offer oral rehydration solutions (Pedialyte) or other clear fluids. Water is okay if there is no vomiting.

If she is at the stage where she is eating solids
- Don't worry if she doesn't want to eat for several days. She'll lose weight but regain it when her appetite returns.
- Avoid dairy foods and fruit juices, as they may exacerbate the loose stools.
- Offer a well-balanced diet, but know it's okay if your child doesn't want to eat anything at all.
- Most important: lots of fluids will prevent a trip to the emergency room!

Call your doctor if
- Your baby doesn't urinate at least three times in twenty-four hours.
- There is blood in her stool.
- Your baby is inconsolable or has a fever for more than seventy-two hours.

CHAPTER 7

CRY

What's All the Fuss About?

∙ ∙

Half of my patients call because they're worried that their child never cries. The other half complains that their baby cries all the time. If you fall into the first group, I wouldn't tell any of your friends who have new babies, because they'll be jealous. That's because crying is one of the most basic things a baby does—and yet it's one of the most common concerns new parents have.

Babies cry for all sorts of reasons. But until you learn to figure out what each cry means and how to respond, you may feel exasperated and helpless. In this chapter, I'll demystify crying so that everything tear-related becomes perfectly clear, including:

- Why babies cry
- How to decipher what different cries mean
- Crying times of the day
- Colic
- Crying to get what she wants

I'll also offer my Common Sense Parenting Diagram of Crying so that you'll be able to track the trail of your baby's tears.

Why Babies Cry—*and How Can I Tell What Different Cries Mean?*

Crying is your child's primitive way of communicating. Yes, it would be much easier if she could just tell you that she's hungry or needs her diaper changed, but that would take all the fun out of parenting. So what you need to do is become a translator of your baby's cries. There are different cries for different emotions and needs. Infants cry when they're hungry, tired, sick, in pain, cold, hot, yearning for attention, or for no reason at all, and each cry tends to have its own characteristics. Over time, you'll be able to tell one type of cry from another. Like everything else in life, the more you practice the better you'll get.

Hungry cries often start with a whimper, then escalate to a longer, louder, repetitive wail. Painful cries, on the other hand, are usually high-pitched, piercing outbursts that make you snap to attention as you would when hearing an ambulance siren. Since your baby's desperate cries can sometimes bring you to tears, I've put together a Common Sense Parenting Diagram of Crying that will help you decipher what your infant needs so that you can appropriately spring into action. You'll notice that each section of the diagram is organized around the times of day when you're most likely to hear particular cries: random times, after meals, and early evening.

Crying at Random Times

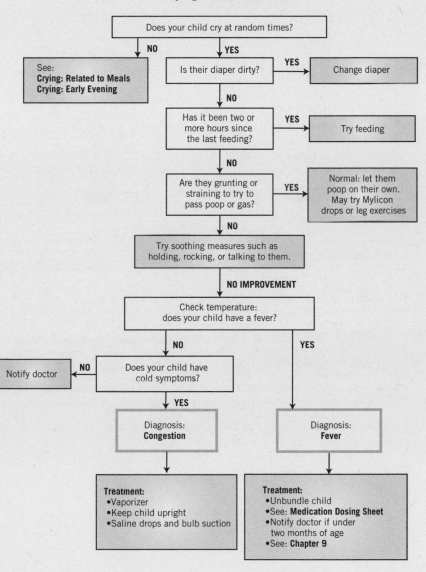

Crying Related to Meals

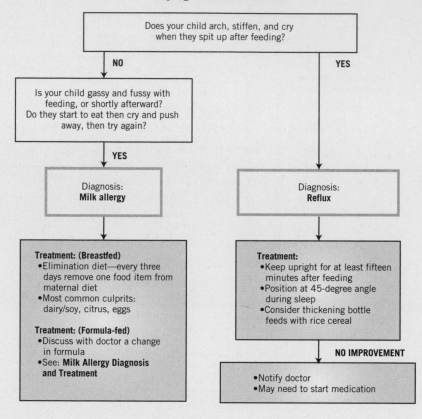

Does your child arch, stiffen, and cry
when they spit up after feeding?

NO   **YES**

Is your child gassy and fussy with
feeding, or shortly afterward?
Do they start to eat then cry and push
away, then try again?

YES

Diagnosis:
Milk allergy

Diagnosis:
Reflux

Treatment: (Breastfed)
- Elimination diet—every three
days remove one food item from
maternal diet
- Most common culprits:
dairy/soy, citrus, eggs

Treatment: (Formula-fed)
- Discuss with doctor a change
in formula
- See: **Milk Allergy Diagnosis
and Treatment**

Treatment:
- Keep upright for at least fifteen
minutes after feeding
- Position at 45-degree angle
during sleep
- Consider thickening bottle
feeds with rice cereal

NO IMPROVEMENT

- Notify doctor
- May need to start medication

Crying in the Early Evening (Two Weeks to Three Months of Age)

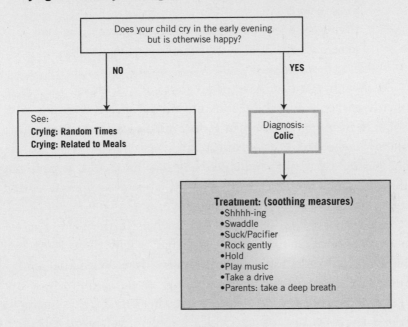

What If My Baby Is Inconsolable?—Colic

"Colic" is the term that describes the inconsolable crying of an infant in the first couple months of life. The dreaded "C" word is one of the most exasperating experiences new parents face. Trying to soothe an infant who cries for hours on end with seemingly nothing wrong with her would drive any parent to tears—and, in fact, it does. So what's going on with a baby who cries even though she's not hungry, wet, tired, or lonely?

There have been many hypotheses about the cause of colic: from gas to reflux to allergies to the notion that a nine-month gestation is too short and infants are just born too early. However, studies have yet to find a single cause of colic. Although we still don't know the cause, there are a few facts about colic that contribute to our understanding of it:

- Colic usually begins around three weeks of age and ends around three months of age.

149

- Colic occurs at least three times a week and lasts for at least three hours a day.
- Crying episodes usually occur in the early evening and are sometimes described as the infant's "witching hours."

Although you may have heard that colic is caused by a milk allergy, gas, or reflux, these ailments are not interchangeable with colic. If an infant cries because of a milk allergy, she has a milk allergy; if she cries because of gas, she has gas; if she cries because she has reflux, she has reflux. A baby may have colic as well, but these ailments are not the cause of it. Colic is a separate entity: inconsolable crying with seemingly no cause.

So, what do I think causes colic? I believe there are a number of factors that cause colic, and that is why there is no one remedy that works for every baby, every time. With that said, I believe that a major factor is emotional stress. Think of how you feel at the end of the day after a harrowing plane trip. Your flight was delayed because of a technical problem, you were forced to wait in your seat where hot air was blowing out of the vents and the cabin was boiling. The stench of recycled air and sweat filled the cabin. The sound of the airplane's engine drowned out your ability to think straight and gave you a headache. On top of that the person sitting next to you invaded your space and jockeyed for the arm rest. You couldn't stretch your legs because there was too little space in coach, the only section you could afford. And if all of that wasn't bad enough, a screaming baby in the row across from you and a two-year-old in the seat behind you kept kicking your seat. Now, how do you feel? Pretty stressed, right?

If a simple airline flight can ruin your day, think of how a day full of stress could affect a newborn baby. It makes sense that the accumulation of all the stresses in a baby's day can result in colic. Colic starts in the early evening because stress builds up all day and comes to a head at night. It begins when a baby is three weeks old because up until that point the infant tends to be sleeping a lot, tuned out, and unaware of her surroundings; and it usually ends when the baby is three months old because at that stage she can more easily filter out the negative stimuli.

150

Interestingly, colic seems to appear primarily in first-born babies. I almost never hear parents complain of colic with their subsequent children. Why? Maybe parents can cope with the colic itself much better. Or maybe with the second child and those that follow, parents can deal better with the stress associated with a newborn, which results in a more serene environment and less stress on the baby.

I remember new parents who came to the office with the concern that their newborn was having problems breathing. During the visit, the infant looked around the room while lying comfortably in his mother's arms. All of a sudden the mother shouted, "Did you hear that?" I was confused, because I didn't hear anything. The mom said, "There it is again," and was practically in tears. She then bounced her son up and down chanting, "You're okay, sweetie! You're okay!" Meanwhile the baby was happy and alert. I watched more closely and realized that the upsetting sound the mother had referred to was the baby's cooing. I reassured her that her son was fine and that what he was doing was absolutely normal. It seems that these parents were always worried about this baby—whether it was a groan, a sneeze, or a hiccup. They were constantly checking on him and waking him up to see if he was okay. The infant couldn't do anything without the family worrying. And guess what? This baby experienced several months of colic. While this may seem like an extreme case, I believe that the parents' anxiety caused their infant to be stressed, which in turn brought on colic.

A baby's stress may be caused by overly anxious parents, but they are not necessarily the only source. Others may include: a dog that won't stop barking, an older sibling who constantly pokes and prods the sleeping infant, extended family members who hover over the baby in an attempt to be helpful.

Think about how you feel when someone is always breathing down your neck, or when everything around you is chaotic. Everyone needs some downtime. Everyone needs to go to their "peaceful place" once in a while to get away from the hustle and bustle of daily life, and infants are no different. That is why some of the best remedies for colic involve soothing measures that mimic the

151

infant's peaceful place. Since babies don't have a lot of life experience to draw from, the most soothing memory is of their time in the womb. Here are some remedies for colic that draw on experiences of being in the womb:

- Swaddle the baby tightly in a cozy blanket, which mimics the warm, cozy intrauterine environment.
- Make a *shhhh*-ing sound, which mimics the sound of blood flowing through the mother's womb. This is the sound the infant heard on a daily basis. It's like white noise.
- Lay the baby on her side and rock her gently back and forth in a large pendulous arc. This mimics the experience of being in the womb and being rocked back and forth with the mother's movements.

Just as adults are not all soothed by the same relaxation methods, not every infant responds to the same soothing measures. Some adults like to sit in a quiet place to relax while others may want to blast rock music to calm their nerves. When it comes to your baby, finding the right way to soothe her may require a little trial and error. Here are just a few suggestions:

- Do some vacuuming in the next room. The monotonous sound of a vacuum cleaner may be calming for your baby.
- Place her in her car seat and put her on top of the clothes dryer so that she hears the humming and feels the warmth of the machine.
- Take her for a drive around the block.
- Play a lullaby CD or some oldies rock music—or sing to her.

My daughter would immediately stop crying if we sang her name to the Mickey Mouse theme song: A-U-B . . . R-E-Y, G-R-A-C-E, Aubrey Grace. . . . Whatever works, stick with it. Remember, there is no one magic remedy to help a baby stop crying, so find the ones that work for your child.

What About Remedies for "Nervous Stomach"—Do They Help Colic?

There are certain remedies that help to soothe an infant's nervous stomach. Again, these do not work for every child with colic because gastrointestinal problems are not always a factor. Still, after a stressful day, just as your stomach is "tied up in knots," often a stressed-out infant will be similarly affected. You may reach for a cup of herbal tea to calm your stomach, and some parents of colicky babies find that the following remedies can be similarly beneficial to a fussy infant:

- Mylicon drops (simethicone)
- Gripe water
- Hyland's Colic Tabs
- Chamomile tea

Mylicon drops are like Gas-X for babies. While gas alone is not the cause of colic, such remedies may help to alleviate some of the contributory symptoms. Gripe water and Hyland's Colic Tabs are homeopathic remedies that may be given to your infant several times a day to help soothe her upset stomach. Similarly, chamomile tea may be calming as well. Place a half to one ounce of warm (not hot!) chamomile tea in a bottle with a pinch of sugar. The quantity does not really matter, but it has no nutritive value so you don't want it substituting for normal feedings. It may not help, but it's worth a shot.

During my pediatric training, pediatricians in private practice used to visit our hospital to give us lectures on common ailments they've seen and possible remedies. When they talked about colic and the unproven remedies they would try, I would scoff. *How dare they give a child something that is not medically proven and most likely has no benefit?* Then, when I started in private practice, parents would tell me that their child would cry for hours on end and they didn't know what to do. I found myself suggesting some of the same remedies I had learned about during my training. Sometimes those remedies were helpful, and sometimes they weren't. Since there was no harm in trying these things, I figured my patients deserved to know about them.

153

Also, I had gone through a personal experience—relating to something much more serious than colic—in which a harmless unproven remedy seemed to have a beneficial affect. When I was in medical school, my dad was diagnosed with lymphoma. At that time, they told him that he had a poor prognosis and not many good treatment options. He went through chemotherapy, radiation, and experimental drugs and finally went into remission. He believes that his cancer was cured by his daily glass of green tea, and who am I to say that it wasn't? I'm just happy he's cured.

Although the remedies for colic are not medically proven, they don't hurt, and they may help. Half of my patients say they are worthless while the other half usually find some success with at least one. Perhaps that success is the result of the placebo affect or the calming affect of the sweet-tasting remedy. Or maybe the particular remedy they used relieved their baby's nervous stomach.

Are You Saying My Baby's Colic Is My Fault?

No, it's not your fault. And I know that some parents of colicky babies out there have been rubbed the wrong way by this chapter. You may be thinking, "How dare he blame me for my child's colic!" My point here is not to blame you, but to find ways to minimize stress in order to help your infant. Colic is probably the result of a genetic predisposition as well as an environmental trigger—in this case stress. But this is not to say that there aren't stress-free households that have colicky babies, as well as stressful environments that are home to easygoing infants. So relax, don't blame yourself, and look to the soothing remedies that work best for your child.

Common Sense Bottom Line

Try to minimize stress in the home in order to decrease your baby's risk of colic. If colic is a problem, experiment with soothing remedies until you find one or more that do the trick. And know that the colic will be gone around three months of age.

Daddy vs. Doctor—Cry, Baby, Cry

Fortunately, Aubrey was not a colicky baby, but there were definitely times she needed to be consoled. When she cried as an infant, we tried the "by the book" remedy: swaddling her tightly. But when we did this, she'd become angry and kicked the blanket away.

Aubrey taught me something fundamental about babies and their personalities. I've learned that the expression "I was just born that way" is actually very true. I remembered that in most of Aubrey's ultrasounds, she had her arms above her head. It made me realize that whatever position a fetus is in while in the womb is likely a soothing position. It makes sense that someone who'd been used to that position in the womb would then feel comforted in that position as a baby. Most nights Aubrey slept with her arms above her head, and any attempt to hold them down in the traditional, swaddling position meant a screaming fit. The book said it was supposed to be soothing, but not for her. When we put a blanket over her while she was sleeping, she would kick it off; and if we put socks on her feet she would rub her feet together until they came off.

The moral to this story: every child is different, so follow her cues when it comes to soothing her . . . and don't forget to check her ultrasound for clues.

Crying to Get What She Wants

Very early on, infants know what they want and how to get it. Most often it's a matter of them training us rather then us training them. During the first four months, the basic advice is to do whatever your baby needs you to do whenever she needs you to do it. You cannot spoil her. Her cries are her way of communicating to you that she needs something, and she needs it now—food, **155** a fresh diaper, a mom's or dad's arms to be rocked or soothed in, sleep, or perhaps something to ease a pain she's having. In those first four months your baby is learning that the world is a safe place because you immediately respond to her needs whenever she cries.

After about four months, if her need isn't an urgent one, we can allow a baby to cry a little longer without rushing to attend to her. (Obviously, if she's sick or in pain, you should go to her when she cries.) Although comforting and holding your baby are still important, as she gets older it is also important that she has her own downtime to relax, explore, and self-soothe. And it's worthwhile to teach her that crying for something inessential is not always the way to go. It is perfectly okay, for instance, to say to an eight-month-old who is crying for you to pick her up, "Mommy is busy right now. I'll be there in a second." This teaches her to self-soothe and reinforces the idea that she will not always get what she wants the instant she wants it simply by screaming louder and longer.

If she's crying because she wants to play with something that's dangerous or inappropriate, offering an alternative will usually do the trick. If she's upset because you took away the fork she grabbed from the table, offer her a wooden spoon. If she's angry and crying because she can't play with the hardback novel you're reading, give her the soft cloth baby book she can teethe on in peace.

Babies need our attention, and crying is one way to get it. But if you give her your love and attention when she's not crying, she will learn that she doesn't always have to cry to get what she needs, and if you don't jump to attention every time she wants the slightest little thing, you allow her to learn to self-soothe.

CHAPTER 8

GROW
Developmental Milestones

· ·

Every parent worries about her child's growth and development, especially in the first year. Is she tall enough, heavy
enough, talkative enough for her age? Why isn't she sitting
up, rolling over, crawling, walking, dancing yet? Such high anxiety stems from the fact that we tend to compare our babies to
other babies—a friend's or neighbor's child, a niece or nephew, a
classmate at the Mommy and Me class. Kevin already smiles, but
Heather doesn't. Zack sips from a cup so why can't Zoe? Suzie
was walking at eleven months, why hasn't Johnny started yet?
My commonsense answer is that a child's development isn't like
an elevator with designated floors ("Sixth floor: six months old.
Time to sit up!"). It's more like an escalator that moves on a continuum.

Some books on childhood development tell you what a child
should be doing at a particular age, like crawling at eight months
or walking at one year. But what if your child is not doing those
things at that age? Should you be concerned? Usually, the answer
is no. I am not concerned if a child is not doing what "the book"
says she should be doing at that age, as long as she's heading in that
direction. For example, it is absolutely normal if your one-year-old
is not walking yet but instead pulls up to stand and moves around
(something she wasn't doing a few months before). As long as she's
making progress, she's doing fine.

157

I have organized this chapter according to what you can expect along the continuum of a child's development, rather than what *should* be happening at a specific time. I'll discuss your baby's development in the same way that I give advice in my office: what you might expect as you look ahead to the next few months. I'll explain what you can do with your infant to encourage age-appropriate development, as well as what you should be monitoring in order to keep her safe.

I'll also debunk some common myths about developmental milestones that can cause parents to either worry needlessly or get their hopes up mistakenly. In the latter category, let me assure you now that your baby's large head will not guarantee her a Harvard admission, nor will his 90th percentile height ranking assure him a basketball scholarship.

At the end of the chapter, we'll talk about teething and when to expect your baby's teeth.

So here we go. Let's talk about your child's developmental progress by breaking down what you can expect during these *approximate* stages along the continuum:

- around two weeks to two months
- around two to four months
- around four to six months
- around six to eight months
- around eight to ten months
- around ten to twelve months
- around one year old—and beyond

What to Expect from Around Two Weeks to Two Months

During this time your infant relies on you for everything, and for most of the twenty-four hours in a day she will simply eat, sleep, and poop. But she'll do some other things as well. She'll lie on her back and flap her arms and legs like a turtle caught upside down. Her vision is very blurry, and she sees best at a distance of about six to twelve inches. Still, she recognizes your shape, smell, and voice from across the room. Don't be surprised if she appears to stare right through you. She may even look cross-eyed from time to time. (If she looks cross-eyed all the time, or still appears cross-eyed after three to four months of age, she should be evaluated by an ophthalmologist.) You may notice that your baby smiles in her sleep or with gas, but not in response to you. That's okay—it's still nice to see her smile. As for her voice, it will make its appearance as you quickly begin to decipher her cries.

Your baby's hands will be clenched tightly in a fist, and if you place your finger in her palm, she will grasp it reflexively. When she's on her stomach, you'll notice that she has trouble lifting her head, but she will often turn it to one side and lay there. If she does lift her head, it will be only briefly, then it will fall back to the ground with a thump.

As your child approaches six to eight weeks old, she may start cooing to express herself, and smiling in response to your voice or a face that you make. This is called a *social smile* and is the first sign that your infant can see. She will start tracking movements briefly—not all the way across the room, but a shorter distance. She may look at you as you move a short distance, then jerk her head and attention in a different direction.

Don't expect her to respond to your voice when you call her name or clap your hands. If she does, great. But if she doesn't, that's just as normal. Some infants can sleep through a train passing by while others startle when a pin drops.

When your baby is on her stomach she may be able to lift her head about 45 degrees off the ground for brief periods. Her hands will still remain clenched and you will still notice her stare blankly into space and go intermittently cross-eyed.

Common Sense Bottom Line

How to encourage age-appropriate development:

- *Tummy time: Two weeks of age is a good time to start tummy time, which helps build neck and back muscles. When your infant is awake, place her on her stomach on a firm surface at least once a day. The amount of time is up to her. If she starts crying after fifteen seconds or fifteen minutes, pick her up. Tummy time also helps to get her used to being on her stomach so that when she starts rolling over she won't cry for you to get her out of that position. Also, being on her stomach occasionally decreases the risk of developing a flat head.*
- *Give her lots of attention: Talk and sing to her. If she cries, comfort her. If she's hungry, feed her. There's no way you can "spoil" your baby at this age.*
- *Offer her objects to look at and touch.*
- *Play tracking games by moving your face and toys back and forth.*

Safety Tips

- Make sure to always put your child to sleep on her back to prevent SIDS. Avoid soft bedding, pillows and blankets, and smoking.
- Avoid crowded areas where your child has a greater chance of being exposed to sick people. Have everyone who comes in contact with your baby wash their hands or use an anti-bacterial hand cream like Purell.
- Car seats should be in the backseat facing to the rear until your child is two years old or outgrows their car seat. This recommendation by the AAP is based on research that showed that children under the age of two are five times safer in a crash and seventy-five percent less likely to die or be severely injured if they remain rear facing until the age of two.
- Make sure your water heater is set to less than 120 degrees Fahrenheit to avoid scalding burns.

Baby Myths

"Joint cracking is abnormal": You may notice that when you lift your infant or move her arms and legs, you hear her joints crack. This is especially common with large joints such as the knees and shoulders and is absolutely normal and happens because an infant's joints are not fully fused yet. As long as she continues to move her extremities after you hear them crack (which she will), there is nothing to worry about.

"Swaddling affects development": Swaddling does not affect your baby's hips, nor does it prohibit motor milestones such as crawling or walking. You can swaddle your child anytime she is sleeping, which in the first couple of months may be several hours a day. Parents often ask at what age they should stop swaddling their infant. My answer: follow her cues. If swaddling puts her to sleep quickly, then keep swaddling. Usually around four months of age children want to roll over or move around, so they fight being swaddled or wake up unswaddled. Take that as a cue to stop swaddling her. On the other hand, if she loves it, you can swaddle her as long as she likes.

What to Expect from Around Two to Four Months

The transition from two months to three to four months old is my favorite developmental change in the next twenty-one years. Up to this point your child has been a little bit of a lump on a log—no offense. Then, at three to four months of age, your infant starts to interact with you more frequently and you will start to feel like you are really getting something back from her. Three huge changes occur to improve this interaction:

- *Vision improves:* Your infant's vision improves from legally blind at birth, 20/200 to 20/800, which means she could not read the big E on the eye chart, to 20/60 by four months of age (close to driving vision, though I do not recommend that just yet). At about three months old, your infant may start tracking 180 degrees horizontally as you walk across a room, then start vertical tracking by four months old. All of a sudden she will love looking around the room and following movements such as the figures dangling from her mobile.

- *Vocalizations increase:* Your infant's cooing will start to transition into high-pitched squeals and screaming. These pterodactyl sounds don't signal that she's hungry or hurt or sick. Instead, they are evidence that she is finding her voice for the first time. She will scream just to scream and express herself. She may also start to giggle or come out with a full guttural laugh.

- *Head, neck, and upper-body strength improves:* This may lead to rolling over. Rolling from stomach to back usually happens first by accident because all the infant has to do is lift her head and lean; the weight of her head propels the rest of her body over. You may see this on and off between two to four months of age or even by accident in the first month of life. Rolling from back to stomach is harder because she has to be strong enough to roll over her arms and elbows, which act like kickstands. This usually doesn't happen until after four months old.

With this newly developed strength come new risks, so remember, never leave your child alone on anything off the ground. It only takes a second for her to roll off.

To test your infant's upper-body strength you can try two maneuvers:

1. Lay her on her back and gently pull her up to a seated position.
2. Hold her prone in your hands like you are imitating Superman.

Notice her posture when you do each of these things, because it will change as she gets older.

At around two months old, you'll see that her head lags all the way as you pull her to a seated position, so you'll need to support her head even when she's sitting. When you hold her in a prone position, her head and legs will droop most of the time.

At around three months old, her head will lag until she is just about in a seated position, then she will be able to hold her head up (although a little wobbly) when she is sitting, with a little body support from you. When you hold her in a prone position, she'll keep her head up above her shoulders, but her legs will still droop a little below her body.

At around four months old, she will lead with her head as you pull her to a seated position and hold her head up with just a little body support from you when seated. In the prone position, she'll hold her head up high and legs straight with her body or even arched above her body like Superman or Superwoman.

Now that your child can sit with support, this is a good age to introduce objects such as the Bumbo chair, Exersaucer, or Jumperoo, in which your infant can sit or stand with help . . . and play!

Daddy vs. Doctor—Rolling Over

Even though I talk to my patients every day about not leaving their baby alone for a second, I had to learn this lesson firsthand. I was watching my daughter while my wife was in the other room. Aubrey was five months old and had just realized the joys of rolling over. I placed her on the couch with the ottoman abutting our L-shaped couch, so she had plenty of room to move around. I walked away to get the TV remote and heard a thump.

I looked back at the couch but my daughter was gone. There was an airy silence; no crying except my wife yelling from the other room, "What was that?" I ran back to the couch to find my daughter lying on her stomach in the six-inch gap between the ottoman and the couch, looking up at me and smiling. Just then, my wife ran into the room in a panic asking, "Did she just fall off the couch?" Avoiding her question, I answered, "Look, she's fine." My wife ran over and picked Aubrey up to make sure she was okay, shot me a look, then got on the phone to announce to all of our family and friends what Dad the pediatrician had just done.

There are several other discoveries that your baby will make during this fascinating period, namely:

- *Finding her center:* Between two to four months of age, babies discover that their arms, legs, and body are attached to them. Before this time, you may have noticed that when your baby was on her back, she would be all splayed out, with her arms and legs outstretched like she was making snow angels. She may have inadvertently got her fist trapped in her mouth or smacked herself in the face. But all that is changing now. At this time, you'll see her put her hands together in front of her face and stare at them perplexed, as if to say, "Ooooh, what are these? Are they mine?" Then she'll start putting her fist in her mouth more deliberately. She may stick her hand in too far at first and gag herself, or try to get both fists in her mouth like a party trick. You will also notice her gnawing on her hands, or punching herself by moving her little fists up and down over her open mouth, which will make her drool. I can predict that a well-meaning relative will tell you this means your baby is teething—but she's not. It's just that drooling and sucking on her hands are among the things that babies at this age do a lot. After all, she's just discovered her hands and her mouth for the first time, and she's having lots of fun exploring and self-soothing.

  As for teething: teeth may erupt between three to six months of age, but usually closer to six months or later. Until you feel the sharp, hard edge of the tooth breaking through the gum, she's not teething. (More on teething at the end of the chapter.)

Just as she discovered her mouth, your infant is going to find other body parts as well. She'll start playing with her ears—rubbing them, twisting them, and pulling them, especially when she's tired. That one neurotic family member (and we all have one) will tell you that your child's pulling on her ear means she has an ear infection. She does not. Again, she's just discovering all her body parts, exploring and self-soothing.

Finally, your baby will start grabbing and pulling her hair (if she has any). It's common, and somewhat comical, to find her arching her back and crying while pulling on her own hair. She's crying because she's unaware that she's the one doing the pulling. Simply release her hand from her hair and you'll see an immediate sense of relief and confusion as she stops crying—and wonders what her hand was doing there.

- *The death grasp:* Around three months of age, many infants start opening up their clenched fists for longer periods of time and grabbing at things. I call this *the purposeless death grasp.* She'll wave her arms in the air and latch on to whatever she comes into contact with. If you have long hair, or are wearing big hoop earrings, glasses, or a necklace, you'll know what I'm talking about.

Common Sense Bottom Line

How to encourage age-appropriate development:

- *Introduce one toy at a time to allow your child to explore and focus on each one. Hold brightly colored toys over her chest as she lies on her back and watch her enjoy reaching up and pulling them close. Good toys at this age include rattles, a soft doll, or a soft picture book.*
- *Let your child play with your fingers.*
- *Respond when she coos by having a conversation.*
- *Continue to encourage tummy time.*

Safety Tips
- Don't hold hot drinks while holding your baby.
- Never leave your child alone on a bed or changing table as she is now old enough to roll off.

What to Expect from Around Four to Six Months

Between four and six months of age your infant's upper-body strength and balance continue to improve, and at around six months of age she may go from sitting with support to being able to sit without support. She won't be able to place herself in a seated position on her own, but if you put her there she will be able to hold herself up without extra support. She may lean forward and hold herself up by leaning her elbows on her legs, then sit more upright as she gets stronger.

Don't be surprised if she holds herself up for just a short period, then falls over to the side when she arches her back or tries to move to get something. She may have the strength and tone to sit without support, but not the patience to do so.

She will also be more aware of her body parts now. After months of putting her hands in her mouth, now she'll go for her feet.

Her dexterity will also improve. The purposeless death grasp will transition into a more *purposeful raking grasp.* Be careful of anything within arm's reach (especially small objects) because your baby will reach for them, rake them in toward her, and put them directly into her mouth. She will also start to transfer objects from one hand to the other.

Although you won't hear any discernible words yet, around six months of age most infants will start screechy-squealy babbling to express themselves.

Also at about six months of age, your child will develop a sense of *object permanence,* meaning she knows that things exist in the world. Prior to this age, if an object was out of sight, it was out of mind. All that has changed now, which is why peek-a-boo suddenly works. Your baby now knows that you exist so when you cover your face, she'll wait in delighted anticipation for you to reappear. Prior to six months of age, when you covered your face with your hands, you simply disappeared from the face of the earth and your baby didn't expect you to reappear. Another example of the difference between these two stages of development is if you show a four-month-old a ball and drop it, she won't look to see where it went because, for her, it literally disappeared. In contrast, a six-month-old will look all over the floor because she knows the ball must have gone somewhere.

Similarly, starting around six months of age you may notice that your infant cries when you leave the room. Her sense of discomfort and fear is called *separation anxiety,* which peaks between six to nine months of age. Before, when you left the room, you were out of sight and thus out of your baby's mind. Now, when you leave the room, she knows you exist and wants you to come back. If your child screams when you leave her with a babysitter or caretaker, don't worry. This is normal behavior. Apologize to whomever you have to leave her with and feel comforted knowing that she may cry when you leave but will be fine five to ten minutes later.

Common Sense Bottom Line
How to encourage age-appropriate development:

- *Try placing your baby in different positions such as on her back, tummy, and sitting with support.*
- *Continue an active dialogue with your child. Give her time to respond to and imitate your actions.*
- *Provide a variety of safe toys and encourage exploration. Press a button or shake a toy and allow time for her to try.*
- *Exersaucers and bouncers are fun at this age.*
- *Walkers are a no-no. They are dangerous and build the wrong leg muscles for walking.*

Baby Myth

"Bouncing or standing her up hurts your infant's legs and back and may delay walking and cause her to be bowlegged": Many parents report that their child loves to stand or be bounced up and down, but they're fearful that this will hurt the baby's legs or

167

back or make her bowlegged. This is not true. All infants are bowlegged to some degree because of their position in utero. Although some people may remember a relative or friend who wore braces to straighten out his legs, you would be hard-pressed to find anyone wearing them today. An infant's bow legs naturally straighten out on their own by twenty-one to twenty-four months of age. At that age, babies actually may become knock-kneed for a couple of years and their legs straighten out again for good. So an infant with bowlegs is usually normal—and bouncing them *does not* cause bowleggedness anyway. As for hurting her, your child will let you know if you are hurting her legs when you stand her up or bounce her.

Common Sense Bottom Line

If she's laughing and smiling, you are not hurting her. If she's crying, she obviously doesn't like what you are doing and you should stop.

What to Expect from Around Six to Eight Months

During this time, three significant changes may occur.

- First, the good news: your baby may start crawling. Now the bad news: your baby may start crawling. As your child's upper-body strength continues to improve, she will be able to sit upright without support for longer periods. When she is on her stomach she will start pivoting around on her belly. If you place her on her stomach facing in one direction, you'll soon find her heading in another. She may start scooting on her belly like an inchworm. At first, she may actually scoot backward; all the while her knees will be pointed outward, perpendicular to her body like a frog. Then around eight months of age she may start to get her knees underneath her, her butt up in the air, and rock on all fours until she figures out how to coordinate her movement forward in a crawl.

Every parent waits eagerly for his child to be mobile. Then, when the crawling begins, they're shocked to find out what it entails for the parents! When our daughter started crawling, my wife and I looked back longingly at how easy it was to take care of a four-month-old. At that age we could plop her on the floor and do tasks around the house without worrying that she was going to hurt herself. Now that she was crawling, we felt like we were professional spotters, chasing her around making sure she didn't choke on the cat's toys or find a stray paper clip lurking in a corner somewhere. As a pediatrician, I realize that development is all about one step, then the next. As a father, as much as I wanted my baby to crawl, once she did, I often longed for that peaceful precrawl period. So, trust me: there is no rush.

- Second, your infant is going to start *hard consonant babbling*, which means using words with hard consonants like "d" and "b" such as "dadada," "bababa," and "mamama." These vocalizations will be indiscriminate, so do not take it personally when she calls the refrigerator "dada." I know there is an unspoken competition between mothers and fathers about which name the infant will say first. So, let me settle the debate. Dads: if your infant says "dada" first, it means your baby likes you better. Moms: don't worry if your baby says "dada" first; it's only because it is easier for her to pronounce than "mama." It doesn't mean she prefers Dad over you.

- Finally, your child's dexterity continues to become more refined. If you thought the raking grasp was dangerous, now it is going to turn into a *claw or pincer grasp*. This means that not only is your child mobile, but now she wants to pick up even the tiniest objects and put them in her mouth. Time to safety proof.

There are other behaviors you may notice as well, including:

- *Stranger anxiety:* Your infant's separation anxiety may turn into stranger anxiety, which peaks between nine to twelve months of age. The phrase is a bit of a misnomer because

169

your baby is going to cry not just with strangers, but with anyone she doesn't see on a regular basis. Warn the grandparents because they always take it the hardest. Don't be surprised when you try to pass the baby to a loving grandmother and your baby bursts into tears. Or screams bloody murder when Grandpa walks into the room. Again, this is a normal developmental phase. If you do have to leave your baby with someone she doesn't see every day, reassure that person that the baby will be fine in ten to fifteen minutes after you leave.

- *Willfulness:* Children around eight months old start expressing their will. I won't call their outbursts temper tantrums yet, but be warned that this may be a preview of the "terrible twos." Parents commonly ask me if it is too early to discipline their child. The answer is, "No, but pick your battles." The more your child gets away with now, the more she will try to get away with later. If she screams to be picked up and you drop everything to do it immediately every time, you are reinforcing the idea that screaming gets her what she wants. If she wants to be held and you can hold her, fine. But if you are busy, it is okay to say, "Honey, Mommy can't pick you up right now," then let her cry a little bit. If she's crying because she wants something dangerous, like a knife, obviously you cannot give it to her— so she'll have to cry. As soon as she starts to calm herself down, that is a good time to pick her up and explain what you did. "Mommy was busy, but now she can hold you," or "You can't have the knife because knives are dangerous, but here is a spoon to hold." Your child may not understand your explanation, but the repetition helps over time. Most important, you are reinforcing the idea that screaming won't get her what she wants, but that when she is calmed down, you will give her the attention she needs.

Don't think for a second that your child does not know what she wants and how to get it. On the other hand, at this age, when you say "No, don't touch that," or "Yes, I like it when you do that," it tends to mean the same thing to your child: you spoke to her and gave her your attention. What's important is to reinforce good behavior by saying such things as "I love it when you play with your blocks so nicely." Or "I like it when we read stories together." Feel free to go over the top with your enthusiastic endorsement of the good things your baby is doing. The more you give her attention in this way, the more your child will seek attention by doing good things.

If she wants something she can't have, distraction works well at this age. Moving to another part of the room or offering her a different object to play with or simply clapping your hands may break a crying fit. On the other hand, if you can ignore the crying—when it's about wanting something she can't have—ignore it. I know this can be very difficult to do, but it will serve you well in the long run.

Common Sense Bottom Line

How to encourage age-appropriate development:

- *Continue giving your infant feedback. Explain to her what she is doing—for example, "Yummm, you're eating peaches."*
- *Continue playing games like peek-a-boo.*
- *Don't be afraid to discipline her in a gentle but firm way, by not giving in when she cries for something she can't have. Allow her to learn that if she screams for what she wants, she won't get it; but if she calms down you will give her the attention she needs.*
- *Reinforce her good behavior by telling her you're pleased when she's doing something positive.*

Safety Tips

Safety proof your home by doing the following:

- Lock up all poisons and dangerous items.
- Put safety lids on all trash cans, including the small ones in the bathroom where such items as disposable razors are discarded. Or place them high enough that your baby can't reach them.
- Put safety locks on toilet seats.

171

- Affix window blind cords to the wall or tie them up (to prevent strangulation).
- Block off stairways and space heaters.
- Put locks on all windows.
- Put plastic covers on all electrical outlets.
- Cover sharp edges of furniture with padding.
- Place your pet's water bowl somewhere where your infant can't reach it (to prevent drowning).

Despite the best safety proofing, your child will probably find something she is not supposed to. I often receive calls from frantic parents whose babies have ingested a dangerous substance that was brought into the home by other people. So get into the habit of taking visitors' bags and purses and placing them up high on a shelf. You don't want to be talking to your friend only to find your child eating something out of her purse—whether it's a medication, a lipstick, or Tic-Tacs. Make sure you have the phone number handy for Poison Control (1-800-411-8080) and keep Children's Benadryl at home in case of an allergic reaction.

Daddy vs. Doctor—Safety Proofing

When Aubrey was six months old, it was time to safety proof our home. I am not what you would call a handyman. That being said, I wanted to try to put up Aubrey's safety gate. I have watched my share of HGTV home improvement shows, so how hard could it be. My wife politely reminded me of my lack of home-improvement skills, but I was determined. After purchasing a safety gate at the local hardware store, I laid out all the parts on Aubrey's floor. I sat down next to Aubrey (my helper) and started to assemble the gate. My wife walked by, smirked, and said sarcastically, "Good luck," and walked downstairs.

As I was sweating, trying to figure out the installation, I heard my wife say, calmly, "You are a wonderful dad." I thought to myself, *Uh-oh, what did I do wrong?* Before I could respond to my wife, she said, "Look at your daughter." I turned and saw Aubrey laying happily on her stomach, kicking her feet and smiling. She was holding three long screws in one hand and the screwdriver in the other. She was also lying on about ten screws I had dumped out of the package. I had been so preoccupied reading the instructions that I stopped paying attention.

I quickly learned my first rule in safety proofing. No matter how much (or little) you safety proof, you have to keep an eye on your child at all times.

Baby Myths

"Skipping developmental milestones, such as crawling, is a problem": You'll probably hear things like, "If your child doesn't crawl, her development will be affected later on." This is not true. It does not matter if your baby skips a milestone to do something more advanced. Certainly, if a child does not crawl because she's too weak or floppy to do so, that would be a concern. But, if an infant skips crawling only to start pulling up to stand, there is absolutely no cause for concern because she is doing something that takes more strength and muscle tone than crawling. Once an infant can do something more advanced, don't worry about what the previous milestone was. Remember, development is on a continuum and you can skip levels. I see a lot of infants skip crawling, especially those who have older siblings. This is because right around the age they could crawl they also realize that they are strong enough to pull up and stand, and they see their older brother or sister running around, so they think, *Hey, why should I crawl when I can get up and move around like them?* Also, infants spend less time on their stomach than ever before because of the back-to-sleep campaign. As a result, many infants do not like to be on their stomach and may skip rolling onto their stomach or crawling simply because they don't like the position—not because they can't.

173

"Quirky behaviors mean your child has autism": Around eight months of age many children begin demonstrating some quirky behaviors. Parents are often concerned because they read or hear that autistic children engage in some of these same behaviors. The fact is, these behaviors are extremely common and absolutely normal at this age, and if your child's development is otherwise progressing, you should not be concerned. The behaviors in question include: head banging, head shaking, and body shaking.

- *Head banging:* There are two types of head bangers. One type bangs to self-soothe and the other does it out of frustration or anger. Repetitive head banging in a calm child is usually a self-soothing behavior. For example, some babies will hit their head back and forth gently against their mattress or crib to help themselves fall asleep. On the other hand, there are babies who will bang their head against a wall or even a hard floor when they are angry. Both types of behaviors are normal.

  In the case of a temper tantrum, you want to make sure that your child is in a safe place and ignore the behavior. I have never seen a baby seriously hurt herself because of a tantrum. She may cause a bump or a bruise, but if she hits her head hard enough to actually hurt herself, she will stop and not do it again. A child who is doing this wants your attention, and if you feed into it, it will prolong the behavior.

- *Head shaking* is another common behavior at this age. Children shake their head back and forth violently like they are shaking their head "No." This is also normal. A baby may do this if she is frustrated or angry, or because it is fun, or because she is receiving attention for doing it.

- *Body shaking:* Some babies tense their body and shake in a behavior I refer to as "the Hulk." A child will flex her arms at 90 degrees, clench her fists and jaw, and shake as if she is posing for the Mr. Universe Pageant. I often see this behavior when a child is sitting in a high chair eating, but it may appear at any time. A baby does this either to get attention or because she likes it; in either case, it is short-lived and nothing to worry about.

Common Sense Bottom Line
Head banging, head shaking, and body shaking are normal behaviors at this age, so ignore them.

What to Expect from Around Eight to Ten Months

Now that your infant is mobile she may want to up the ante. Starting around ten months of age, your child may start pulling up to-stand against objects such as the sofa or her crib gate. Then she may start cruising or moving from one object to the next as she holds on to each object or piece of furniture. She may even let go for a second while she transfers from one object to the next. Or stand up in the middle of the room on her own. Then, once she realizes she is standing without holding on to anything, she'll plop onto her butt. Once a child can pull up to stand and cruise, she has enough muscle strength and tone to walk. It is just a matter of her getting the gumption to do so. If a child can pull up to stand, or walk holding your hand but won't let go, it just means she's cautious. I have seen babies who will walk holding their parent's pinky. Dad's pinky isn't giving the baby any support, but it gives her the confidence to move forward. If Dad removes his finger, she'll fall to the ground.

As for language, there may not be tremendous changes between eight to ten months of age. Your baby will continue to screech and squeal and hard-consonant babble, still indiscriminately.

Common Sense Bottom Line

How to encourage age-appropriate development:

- *Comfort your child when she cries and acknowledge her feelings when she is frustrated.*
- *Ask her questions such as, "Do you want this toy?" wait for her to respond, then give it to her. Such conversations help to develop her socialization, emotional well-being, language, and motor skills.*
- *Encourage her participation in games such as placing a block in the proper hole or building a tower.*
- *Since she may be experiencing some separation anxiety, be reassuring when you leave and tell her you will miss her but that you'll be back.*

Safety Tips

- If you still have bumpers in her crib, take them out. Children at this age are as strong as Mighty Mouse. Even the thin collapsible bumpers can be used as a stepping ladder to vault her out of her crib. Without the bumpers, she may hit her head against the crib and possibly even bruise herself, but this is nothing compared to falling out of the crib.
- Move the crib mattress to the lowest level.

Baby Myth

"Ear pulling means she has an ear infection": Not so, if this is the baby's only "symptom." Parents often come into my office concerned that their child has an ear infection even though the baby is not fussy and doesn't have a cold or fever. I assure them that ear pulling alone is not a sign of an ear infection, but it is a very common self-soothing behavior in babies and typically shows up around eight months of age. So how can you tell if your baby's ear pulling is a self-soothing behavior or an infection?

- If your child is pulling on her ears but is otherwise happy and doesn't have a cold or fever, then it is likely a self-soothing behavior.
- If she's pulling her ears and is fussy, or has a fever or cold, then check with your pediatrician because she may have an ear infection or feel pressure in her ears from a stuffy nose.
- Finally, check the creases behind your child's ears because she may have dry, cracked skin. Dry skin is very itchy and could be causing her to pull on her ears. If the skin behind your baby's ears is cracked, moisturize the area. If the area is also red, you can use 1 percent cortisone cream twice a day to get rid of the inflammation.

What to Expect from Around Ten Months to One Year

You are almost there. Your baby's first birthday is right around the corner, and she almost seems like a teenager with the progress she has made since she was born. She is now very mobile—crawling fast or cruising, maybe even taking a few steps by twelve months of age. Her babbling may not change much; however, some babies will start to discriminate between "mama" and "dada" by a year old. If she doesn't, don't worry; she'll reach that milestone very soon. You may notice that she has a more sophisticated inflection when she babbles, as if she's having a conversation with you in a foreign language. This is a sign of her developing maturity as well. And she probably has a more refined fine pincer grasp, so be sure to hide those small objects!

How to encourage age-appropriate development:

- *When she becomes frustrated, comfort her and acknowledge her feelings.*
- *Continue to engage her in an active dialogue by talking to her, listening to her, and responding to her.*
- *Encourage her to participate in games with you, such as rolling a ball back and forth, clapping and dancing to music, and playing with puzzles.*

What to Expect Around One Year—*and Beyond*

Over the next few months, your child's motor skills will continue to skyrocket. If she's not walking yet, she will be soon; and soon after that, she'll start running. She can already climb up a bookcase if she wants to, so keep a close eye on her. She's likely feeling her new power and anxious to exercise it!

Language development is one of the most interesting changes you'll witness over the next year. Her developing language skills are twofold:

- *receptive language* (what your child understands), and
- *expressive language* (what your child says)

As you would expect, your child is going to understand much more than she can express to you at this point, which is why two-year-olds still have temper tantrums. You may want to think of this particular period of language development in this way: the first half of the year (between one year and eighteen months) is all about understanding, and the second half of the year (eighteen months to two years) is all about speaking.

Between twelve and fifteen months, she may only develop three to five words, and they won't be perfectly articulated. Instead, she will speak in strings of babble with a word such as "ba" for "ball" thrown in. By eighteen months, she may have only ten to twenty spoken words. On the other hand, once your baby is about twelve months old, you will probably notice that she seems to understand much more of what you say to her. The goal by eighteen months of age, even if she is not saying much, is for your child to follow simple commands such as "Go get your shoes," to look when you point at something, to show interest in things like reading a story, and to show interest in other children. Her level of understanding and her attempts at speech indicate that her language skills are expanding. In the second half of the year, you'll see her vocabulary take off.

Common Sense Bottom Line

How to encourage age-appropriate development:

- *Encourage your child to use her words to communicate.*
- *Read to her and play games that involve pretending and imitating, such as a play kitchen or toy telephone.*
- *Narrate your day-to-day actions so that your child learns to put words to the things that she wants or does. For instance, if she goes to the refrigerator and points and grunts, and you know she wants milk, say to her, "Do you want the milk?" then, "Here's the milk."*

Safety Tip
- Keep your child in a rear-facing car seat. If she has outgrown her infant car seat, buy a convertible seat that can be rear facing now and you can convert to a forward-facing position at two years old.

Should He Play for the Celtics or the Lakers?—Height, Weight, and Head Size

Parents can become nearly obsessed with their child's height, weight, and head size, especially if the child's percentiles are in   **179** direct opposition to her parents'. There is no greater joy on the faces of parents who are five feet tall to find that their six-month-old is in the 90th percentile for height. Then there are those parents who want early assurance that their baby will become as bright as they are, which is why two Ivy League graduates hope that their four-month-old's head size (in the 95th percentile) means she'll most certainly attend their alma mater.

Unfortunately, your baby's percentiles do not mean much more than that she is tall or heavy or big-headed *at this particular time in her life*. I don't want to burst anybody's bubble, but your child's height, weight, and head size in the first year of life have no bearing on her future size or shape. In fact, a baby's future height, weight, and head size have more to do with her parents' current height, weight, and head size than her own when she's a baby. It is all about genetics. Short parents usually have children who grow up to be short, and tall parents usually have children who grow up to be tall.

So what do percentiles mean? When your child is measured as a baby, his height, weight, and head size are compared to those of other children the same age and gender. So, if your son falls on the 50th percentile, that means that half the baby boys his age are smaller and the other half are bigger. On the other hand, if your son is on the 95th percentile, it means he is one of the five biggest out of every hundred baby boys. The point is, though, that it doesn't matter if he's on the 5th percentile or the 95th, as long as he is growing and progressing. Also, a child's percentiles may change a lot over the first six months of his life as he falls in line with his genetic predisposition. For instance, two very petite parents may have a twelve-pound baby. However, given the baby's genetic makeup, it's very unlikely he will grow up to be a "hulk." Although that baby may start off at the 95th percentile, his percentile ranking will usually decrease as he grows.

As long as your baby is growing and thriving, there is no need to be concerned with percentiles.

Common Sense Bottom Line

Being a tall baby doesn't guarantee a basketball scholarship, being a heavy baby doesn't determine a future enrollment in Weight Watchers, and having a large head as a baby doesn't mean a free ride to Harvard. So don't worry about percentiles. If your child is growing at a healthy pace, that's all that matters. If she stops growing at a healthy pace, your doctor will look into possible causes.

Stages of Teething and Tooth Eruption

Another exciting milestone in the first year of your baby's life is the arrival of her teeth. Well, it's not always so exciting when she's teething; in fact, she can feel pretty miserable at times. But if you know what to expect, you can put your mind at ease and help her feel more comfortable. The first thing to expect is what I call the *preteething* stage.

I call it preteething because your baby isn't really teething, although she may show all the signs of it, such as drooling, hands in her mouth, and rubbing her gums with her fist. You may feel ridges when you rub your fingers along her gums; however, these are *gum ridges,* not erupting teeth.

You'll know when a tooth is erupting. When you run your finger along your baby's gum (usually the lower one), you will feel the hard sharp edge of the tooth. What we call *teething* is when a tooth is erupting through the gum, causing swelling of the surrounding gum tissue. This inflammation and swelling may cause more drooling, fussiness, and possibly a low-grade fever (nothing over 101 degrees Fahrenheit). A runny nose and watery stools may also be seen with teething.

It may take several weeks for your baby's tooth to fully erupt, and during this time she will find comfort in sucking on her hands or cold teething rings. She may benefit from Tylenol if she's extremely fussy.

Here is a picture of the typical eruption pattern. If your child does not follow this pattern exactly, there is no cause for concern. This is just the most likely scenario.

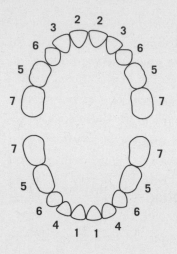

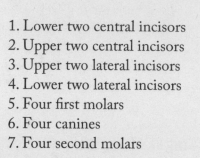

1. Lower two central incisors
2. Upper two central incisors
3. Upper two lateral incisors
4. Lower two lateral incisors
5. Four first molars
6. Four canines
7. Four second molars

Typically, two teeth will erupt about every two to three months. However, don't be concerned if there is a slower or faster pattern. My daughter got her two lower central incisors at around six and a half months of age and did not get another tooth until after her first birthday. Some infants will appear to have a new tooth popping out every couple of weeks, while others may have a long delay between each tooth, then several at once.

Don't worry if your child remains toothless for a while. The upper limit of normal tooth eruption is around eighteen months. This means, in an otherwise healthy infant, I would not do anything but wait for the first tooth until eighteen months of age. At eighteen months, if there are still no teeth, I would order an X-ray to make sure there are teeth in the gums waiting to erupt.

Usually by two years of age it will look like your child has a full mouth of teeth. Actually, she probably has only sixteen out of twenty of her primary teeth. Sometime between the ages of two and two and a half, she'll get her final four primary teeth (the second molars way in the back).

When Should I Start Brushing Her Teeth?

Before she has any. Before your baby has any teeth in her mouth, as early as four to six months old, I suggest that you introduce her to "tooth" brushing. Rub her gums with your fingers or a wet washcloth twice a day. This not only will feel soothing to her, it will also help her get used to you going in her mouth, so she won't fight you when you try to brush her teeth later on.

Once she actually has teeth, you can use a washcloth, finger brush, or toothbrush with or without baby toothpaste. Do not use regular toothpaste (which has fluoride) until your child is able to spit (usually around two to two and a half years old) because you do not want her ingesting too much fluoride. Brushing and wiping down the teeth help to wipe off any residue building up from food or milk and decrease the risk of cavities.

I also recommend that you have her watch you brush your teeth, so that you become a positive role model. Babies love to mimic what their parents do.

Daddy vs. Doctor—Teething

Sometimes my own advice backfires. My daughter had been used to sleeping through the night when one night she woke up several times screaming. Sticking to our guns with the "don't go in and pick her up" advice, my wife and I watched her on the monitor and let her cry. She didn't cry for long, but she was up several times that night crying. She had been fine that day, and I knew she wasn't sick or hungry.

The next morning she woke up and was sitting in her crib smiling as usual, but I noticed she was sucking on her hands. I picked her up and felt her gums and there it was: the edge of her first tooth. She had probably been in pain the previous night, and I felt horrible. I knew I hadn't harmed her, but I had been a bad dad. Obviously, Aubrey was not holding a grudge, but it made me second-guess her crying the next time. Sometimes Dad's intuition should supersede "the rules."

CHAPTER 9

HACHOOO!

Common First-Year Health Concerns

U nless you place your baby in a bubble, she is going to get sick. In fact, children typically contract ten to twelve illnesses within the first two years of life. It isn't a happy thought, but childhood illnesses are very common. Fortunately, most are not serious and we can deal with them fairly easily. Again, the more you know as a parent the better prepared you'll be when your little one wakes up in the middle of the night with a cough or a cold or a fever.

In this chapter, I'm going to help you identify what is going on with your baby when she has certain symptoms or comes down with a specific illness. I'll provide practical advice that will help you and your child get through the night, and I'll let you know what I would be thinking if you were to bring your sick child to my office with a particular medical concern.

I'll also help you to distinguish between something you could handle on your own, a condition that warrants your doctor's attention, and a true medical emergency.

We'll focus on these common first-year health concerns:

- Fever
- Colds
- Croup
- Vomiting

- Hand, foot, and mouth
- The "Slapped cheek" virus
- Roseola
- Rashes
- Wheezing
- Bronchiolitis
- Ear concerns
- Eye concerns

I'll also debunk various myths associated with some of the common illnesses your child may encounter. The less you have to worry about, the better; and untruths are definitely not worth fretting over.

She's Feeling Hot, Hot, Hot—Fever

When children have fever, especially small infants, they look and feel horrible, which can make you worry more than you may need to. Your baby may appear lethargic, her body may shiver, her eyes may roll back, her skin may feel hot to the touch, she may cry or whine and not want to eat. You may even notice that she's breathing rapidly and her heart is racing. These are all normal symptoms of fever—and they'll disappear when the fever goes away. Despite how awful your child may feel and look, fever is actually a good thing.

Fever is the body's normal reaction to an infection. It means your child's immune system is working and the body is trying to fight the infection. The higher temperature creates a less hospitable environment for the infection. Treating the fever does not make the infection go away any quicker. In fact, the only reason we treat the fever is to make your child feel better. If we let her fever persist, it would not hurt her. She would just continue to feel crummy.

So what's the definition of a fever? A fever is defined as a temperature of 100.4 degrees Fahrenheit or greater. A temperature of 99 or 100 degrees is *not* a low-grade fever. It is not a fever at all, contrary to the commonly held belief that anything other than 98.6 means something must be wrong. Actually, our body temperature fluctuates throughout the day and night, so we don't have just one normal temperature. Temperatures of 97, 98, 99, and even 100 degrees may all be normal.

How do you find out if your baby has a fever? The best way to take her temperature in the first two months is with a digital rectal thermometer. A rectal temperature is the most accurate, and accuracy is important because a temperature of 100.3 degrees Fahrenheit versus 100.4 degrees Fahrenheit in a child under two months old is the difference between doing nothing and taking her to the emergency room for a battery of unpleasant tests to rule out infection.

After two months of age you can use a digital axillary (underarm) thermometer. Because your child has had her first set of vaccinations at this age and is better able to handle infection, she probably won't need to be taken to the emergency room for fever. Whether her temperature is 101 or 104, you can treat the fever at home by giving her Tylenol (acetaminophen) or Motrin (ibuprofen) after the age of six months. A dosing sheet for common medications used to treat fever can be found on page 266.

As a parent, I know that when your baby is burning up with fever, it can make you very anxious. However, as a doctor, I am actually more concerned with four things:

1. The number of consecutive days your child has had a fever
2. Whether or not her fever responds to the proper dose of fever-reducing medication
3. How your child looks when she does not have a fever
4. The age of your child (if under two months)

If your child is more than two months of age, regardless of whether her fever is 101 or 105, you need to treat it with the proper medication and wait to see how she responds. She may not be her normal cheery self, but she should be in better spirits once her fever goes down.

Why should you not be alarmed by a high fever? Viruses tend

to cause some of the highest fevers in children; however, a temperature of 105 does not mean that your child has a more serious infection. Typically, viral fevers subside after about seventy-two hours. The other symptoms, if there are any, may persist for several weeks. Once the fever goes down, it is a sign that the infection is going away and that your child is getting better, even if the other symptoms remain.

Viruses can cause colds and fever, but they can also cause fever without any other symptoms. When I see a child who has a fever and no other symptoms, I explain to the parents that usually one of three scenarios may occur:

1. The fever may come and go for about seventy-two hours and go away without any other symptoms developing. In this case, we assume that the child had a viral fever and she is now over it.
2. Your child may start with a fever, then develop other viral symptoms such as a cough and cold a day or two later. These symptoms will usually persist after the fever goes away.
3. The fever may subside and a day later your child breaks out in a rash, a viral infection called *roseola*, which will be discussed later in the chapter.

Fever without symptoms, especially in younger infants, may also be a sign of a bacterial infection such as a urinary tract infection (UTI), so your pediatrician may want to test her urine or blood.

Remember, *the number of days that your child has had a fever is more important than how high her fever is*. If your child has had a fever for more than three days, or the fever-reducing medication does not lower it, you should check in with your doctor. But don't panic. A fever for seventy-three hours or more is rarely a cause for alarm. You simply want the pediatrician to determine whether your baby may still have a virus, or if she has developed a secondary infection such as an ear infection or a bacterial infection such as pneumonia or UTI. Whatever the possible cause, after three days of a fever, call your doctor.

Fever Myths

"Fever causes brain damage": False. Fever does not cause brain damage. Fever is a good thing; it is your body's normal response to an infection.

"A high fever will cause a seizure": False. Actually, febrile (fever-related) seizures are due to how fast a child's temperature rises, not how high it is. Many children who have such seizures did not have a temperature before the seizure occurred. Rather, their temperature rapidly rises from normal to perhaps 101 and that is what causes them to seize. But this is a rare occurrence. Think about how many times you have had a fever in your life and how many times it has caused you to have a seizure. Exactly.

"The best way to lower a temperature is by alternating between Tylenol and Motrin": Not really true, but there's some confusion on this one so let's try to clear it up. First of all, Tylenol and Motrin are different medicines but they're equally effective in reducing fever. The only difference in their effectiveness is in how long each lasts. Motrin (ibuprofen) lasts six hours, while Tylenol (acetaminophen) lasts four hours. When taking either one, you need to wait the specified amount of time between doses: four hours between doses of Tylenol, and six hours between doses of Motrin.

Where does the alternating come into the picture? Since Motrin and Tylenol are two different medicines, you can give your baby one medication during the interval while you're waiting to take the next dose of the other—if your baby's fever hasn't gone down. For example, if you give your child Motrin and her fever doesn't subside or returns before the six hours are up, you can give her Tylenol in the interim. If you started with Tylenol and her fever doesn't subside or returns before the four hours are up, you can give her Motrin in the interim. Because they are different medicines there is not a specific amount of time that you have to wait between the Motrin and the Tylenol. Just make sure to give one the necessary time to work before you try the other. *But do not alternate the two medications just to alternate.* If the Tylenol or Motrin keeps the fever down the whole time, avoid the confusion and stick to one medication. I usually recommend Motrin for fevers at night because it tends to last longer, which may help your baby get a better night's rest.

Common Sense Facts: Fever
What Is Fever?
- Fever is your body's normal reaction to an infection—it is a good thing.
- Fever is a temperature of 100.4 degrees Fahrenheit or higher.
- A temperature of less than 100.4 is normal and does not need to be treated.

What Is the Best Way to Take a Baby's Temperature?
- Rectal temperatures are the most accurate and should always be used in babies under two months of age.
- An underarm temperatures in children older than two months may be used.
- Ear thermometers are notoriously inaccurate and should not be used.

Should I Be Afraid of a Fever?
- *No!*

- Fever, whether it is 101 or 105, will not cause brain damage and will not hurt your child.
- How she looks, acts, and feels when she does not have fever is more important than the number on the thermometer or how she looks when she has a fever.

Will Treating My Child's Fever Make the Infection Go Away?
- No, but it will make her feel better in the interim.

What Medicines Can I Use to Treat a Fever?
- Children younger than six months of age can be given Tylenol (acetaminophen) every four hours as needed.
- Children over six months of age can be given Tylenol every four hours or Motrin (ibuprofen) every six hours as needed.
- Tylenol and Motrin are two different medicines. Therefore, one medicine can be given between doses of the other medicine—if, and only if, the child's fever doesn't go down before her next dose of the first medicine.
- Tylenol and Motrin take approximately thirty minutes to an hour to work. Give the medicine time to work. See page 266 for a dosing chart.

Call Your Doctor If
- your baby is younger than two months of age and has a fever of 100.4 or higher.
- your child (of any age) has a fever that persists longer than seventy-two hours.
- your child's fever does not respond to Tylenol or Motrin.

It's as Common as They Say—Colds

The common cold is called common for a reason. Whether your child is in day care, plays with other children, has an older sibling, or just sits at home alone, she will get many colds throughout her childhood, especially in the winter. It's not that there's anything wrong with her immune system; it's just that the more she's exposed, the more infections she will contract. The good thing is that colds are usually short-lived (although they can last up to three weeks), but sometimes their symptoms can seem scary and make your child feel miserable. Hang in there! We've all had colds and lived through them, and so will your baby.

What causes a cold? Colds are caused by viruses and can be spread by coughing, sneezing, or touching. It's important to remember that viruses and bacteria are not the same, even though they both cause infection. Antibiotics kill bacteria, *not* viruses. So antibiotics are not an appropriate medicine for a cold. Unfortunately, no remedy will make a viral infection go away more quickly. All you can do is make your child feel better until the infection runs its course.

A cold may be accompanied by a runny or stuffy nose, coughing, sneezing, fever—or none of the above. Sometimes the only symptom is a fussy infant. Since your child prefers to breathe through her nose, nasal congestion makes it difficult for her to feed and breathe at the same time. Also, since she spends a lot of time lying on her back, especially at night, mucus drips into the back of her throat, making it hard for her to sleep and breathe. So expect your baby's cough to be at its worst at night and first thing in the morning.

Although you may reach for the Nyquil when you have a cold, over-the-counter cold remedies have not proven to be effective in children under the age of four, and they can even cause death from overdose.

So what can you do to alleviate your baby's symptoms? Here's what I suggest:

1. Run a humidifier or vaporizer in her room to add some moisture to the air and loosen up her congestion. I recommend a cool-air vaporizer (or humidifier; they both add moisture to the air). It doesn't matter if the moisture is warm or cold; however, I recommend a cool-air vaporizer for safety reasons. With the warm one, there's the risk of older children spilling the hot water on themselves and getting burned. As for menthol rubs or placing something in the humidifier like Vicks, it is not recommended. Use of these topical salves or vaporizer additives may actually exacerbate breathing problems in infants and young children.

191

2. Elevate your baby's head by placing a wedge under the mattress or under her head so that the mucus can drain better and doesn't stay in the back of her throat while she's sleeping, which will exacerbate her cough.

3. Try holding your baby upright, a position many infants prefer when they're sick.

4. Limit the use of a bulb suction and saline drops. Every time you stick the tip of the bulb in your child's nose you actually cause irritation, inflammation, and more congestion. You won't be able to suck out a lot of mucus anyway because the congestion is farther back in her nasal passageways. Remember, *if you see something and that something is bothering her, you can suck it out. But if you hear it or see it and your baby is not bothered by it . . . leave it alone.*

5. Make sure your baby gets plenty of rest and fluids.

6. Offer your baby more frequent feedings (of breast milk or formula), but she may want smaller amounts at each feeding to accommodate her stuffiness. And don't forget to pause during feedings to give her a chance to take a breath.

Should you call the doctor if you think your child's cold is really bad? I suggest that you *contact your doctor if:*

- your child has a fever for more than seventy-two hours.
- your child shows signs of dehydration.
- your child has problems breathing.

One way to assess dehydration is to monitor your baby's urine output, so check to see that she has at least three wet diapers every twenty-four hours. If she is peeing less than that, a call to the doctor is warranted. If she hasn't been losing a lot of fluids through vomiting or diarrhea, it shouldn't take much to keep her well hydrated. Even if she's only drinking half as much as normal, she is still getting what she needs.

How can you assess if she's having trouble breathing? By how she looks rather than how she sounds. Most infants with a stuffy nose sound horrible. You may even feel her back rattle when she breathes. Despite how she sounds, however, she usually isn't having any problem breathing. Look at her chest. If it is moving fast and hard, as if she just ran the one-hundred-yard dash, and you see all the muscles around her rib cage or neck pulling in, she is definitely having problems breathing and you should notify your doctor. If, on the other hand, she sounds congested but looks comfortable, and her chest looks like it is barely moving, then she isn't having a breathing problem.

As for when it's advisable to take your baby back to day care or Mommy and Me class, or out to run errands: technically, your child may be contagious as long as she has cold symptoms. But if you kept her home under this strict definition, your child wouldn't be able to leave the house all winter. My Common Sense Parenting advice: once it's been twenty-four hours since she's had a fever, she can go back to doing everything that she feels up to doing. So, waiting until she no longer has a fever means that she'll be feeling better and you'll be reassured that the infection is on its way out. Keep in mind, however, early on in an illness when there are heavy secretions (from the eyes, nose, and mouth) children are more likely to transmit the infection. So, waiting a couple of extra days before returning to class may be considerate to other children. Waiting until your child is completely symptom free, however, is not necessary. Actually, it's impossible to tell which children are contagious and which are not. A baby may have no symptoms but be contagious, because the virus in her system hasn't manifested yet. On the other hand, an infant may be coughing for weeks because of the leftover irritation in her lungs, but she's no longer contagious because the infection itself is gone.

Cold Myths

"My child has a very chesty cough, so it must be in her lungs": Not so. Most infants with colds have a wet-sounding cough. This sound does not usually mean that the infection is in her lungs. Since the mucus drips in the back of her throat and pools there, it may sound as if it is in the lungs. Again, it is more important to evaluate how her breathing *looks* than how it sounds.

193

"Green mucus means she has a bacterial infection and needs anti-biotics": False. A square is a rectangle, but a rectangle is not a square. If you have a bacterial infection, you will usually have yellow or green mucus; but if you have yellow or green mucus it does not mean you have a bacterial infection. Yellow or green mucus just means it has been there longer, not necessarily that there is a bacterial infection that needs antibiotics.

"My child already had this infection so she can't get it again": False. You can get different strains of the same virus. Since there are hundreds of viruses and many of them cause similar symptoms, your child may have the same symptoms with a different virus or she may have contracted a virus she's already had. Other than chicken pox, which you only get once, most viruses can haunt your child for a while.

"Since my child and I have the same symptoms and I am on antibiotics, she needs antibiotics, too": Not likely. Most infections in children are viral and do not need antibiotics. Two people may appear to have similar symptoms but may have two different infections. Just because you have been prescribed medication for your symptoms doesn't mean that your child needs the same medication.

"Milk causes more congestion": Not true. Milk only causes congestion if you are allergic to it. If your baby was fine with milk before she got sick, she'll be fine with milk while she's sick. Her appetite will probably decrease because she's not feeling well. Because milk is usually her favorite drink, you wouldn't want to take away the one thing she likes and will keep her hydrated.

Common Sense Facts: Colds
Symptoms of a Cold
- Coughing
- Sneezing
- Runny nose
- Nasal congestion
- Fever

Treatment
- Vaporizer or humidifier
- Steam shower
- Bulb suction and saline drops (sparingly)
- Lots of fluids
- Tylenol or Motrin for fever

What Not *to Give Your Child*
- Children under four years old should not be given over-the-counter cough/cold medicines.

Call Your Doctor If
- your baby's fever persists longer than seventy-two hours or it doesn't respond to the appropriate dose of Tylenol or Motrin.
- your baby has labored breathing.
- your baby has fewer than three wet diapers in a twenty-four-hour period.

The Baby Is Barking!—Croup

Croup is caused by a virus and usually affects children between the ages of six months to six years of age. A child with croup has a cough resembling that of a barking dog or seal. What is scary about croup is that it tends to show up in the middle of the night. A child with croup typically wakes up with a horrible-sounding cough and trouble breathing. Her breathing can sound as if she is gasping for air. This breathing, which is often described by parents as wheezing, is actually called stridor, and this is the result of the virus causing inflammation that narrows her upper airway. Children tend to outgrow croup as their airway grows wider, to the point that a little inflammation from a virus will no longer cause respiratory distress.

My first Common Sense Parenting rule for croup is to *stay calm.* Your barking, distressed baby tends to look and sound much worse than she really is. Here's how I suggest you treat her:

195

1. Run a hot shower in the bathroom with the door closed to get the room warm and steamy. Sit with your baby for five minutes in the steamy bathroom with the door closed. Warm, moist air seems to work best to loosen the mucus, open her upper airway, and stop the coughing.

2. Next, take her outside into the cold night air. I know our parents used to tell us if we went out in the cold we'd get sick, but in this case the cold is a benefit. Cold air actually opens the upper airway and will usually lessen or eliminate your child's breathing problems. As a doctor and a dad, I find this intervention to be the most useful.

3. If you've tried the steam shower and cold night air, and your child is still having problems breathing, get in the car and head to the emergency room. Drive with the windows down and let your child breathe the cool night air. You may find that by the time you arrive at the hospital, the problem has been eliminated and you can turn around and go home. Fortunately, many children who are rushed to the emergency room are better by the time they get there because their parents have already treated them.

The barking cough and breathing difficulty are usually worse during the first few nights of the illness. Croup can also cause a runny or congested nose and a very high fever. Do not be surprised if your child develops a temperature of 103 to 105 degrees Fahrenheit. Remember, don't worry about how high the fever is, just treat it so that your child feels better. With croup, the fever tends to last up to seventy-two hours. If it persists longer than that, or if your child has a history of breathing problems, you should take her to the doctor. She may need a steroid medication called Decadron to decrease the inflammation in her upper airway.

Common Sense Facts: Croup
What Is Croup?

- Croup is a viral illness that causes fever and inflammation of the upper airway.

- When a child has croup, the airway below the vocal cords becomes swollen and narrow. This makes breathing noisy and difficult and causes a tight, barking cough. The cough is usually worse at night.

Who Gets It and How Long Does It Last?
- Children are most likely to get croup between six months and six years of age. After age six, it is not as common because the windpipe is larger, so swelling doesn't cause a problem.
- Some children get croup often.
- Croup can occur at any time of the year, but it is most common in the winter.
- Like any viral respiratory infection it can last for a week, but usually there are two bad nights of barking cough, and three days or fewer of fever.

What Can I Do to Help My Child?
- *Stay calm!* If you stay calm, your child will stay calm and breathe more comfortably.
- Sit with your baby in a steamy bathroom for five to ten minutes. Then take her out into the cold night air if available.
- Turn on a cool humidifier next to her crib.
- Use Tylenol or Motrin to bring down her fever.

Doesn't She Need Antibiotics or Medicine?
- As with other viruses, antibiotics are not an appropriate medicine.
- If your child continues to have labored raspy breathing she may need an oral steroid that your doctor will prescribe.

Should I Take Her to the Doctor or Emergency Room?
- Take her to the emergency room if she is having difficulty breathing even after trying the steamy shower and the cold-air walk/drive.
- If there is a history of breathing problems or prolonged fevers, see your doctor.

197

Vomiting

Most vomiting is caused by a viral infection. It may be present alone or with a combination of symptoms that include diarrhea, fever, fussiness, and poor appetite.

The best way to treat your baby's suspected stomach virus is to do the following:

- Do not give your baby anything to eat or drink for at least thirty to sixty minutes after vomiting. If she vomits in that period, wait another thirty to sixty minutes. If she falls asleep, let her sleep. If she screams for her bottle or something to drink after she throws up, hold off (per above); if you give her the bottle or the breast, she will chug the milk and just throw up again.

- Give her small amounts of clear liquids (Pedialyte, tea, or watered-down juice) to replace the fluids she is losing by vomiting. Start by offering a teaspoon every few minutes, and gradually increase the amount as tolerated. Pedialyte Popsicles are also an effective way to replenish lost fluids.

- Once she is able to tolerate more liquid, you can give her watered-down formula (if she is on formula) or breast milk. If she vomits in the middle of this process, wait another thirty to sixty minutes and start all over again.

- With breast milk or formula feedings, make sure you pace the feedings by giving her smaller amounts more frequently. And give her frequent breaks during each feeding.

- *Do not* give her plain water. Water lacks the sugar and electrolytes, such as sodium and potassium, that your baby is losing when she vomits. Water may actually increase the vomiting.

Your baby's vomiting will usually be worst in the first twenty-four hours, but it may continue sporadically for seven to ten days. Within that time period, your child may vomit more some days than others. She may skip a couple of days, then start vomiting again. The virus didn't go away and come back, it's just that the symptoms may wax and wane throughout the ten-day course.

If your child is at the eating-solids stage but doesn't want to eat for several days, don't worry! Most children have intermittent abdominal pain with a stomach virus and don't feel like eating. Yes, she may lose a little weight, but she will regain it once she's feeling better—and she *will* feel better, trust me.

Common Sense Bottom Line
- *Avoid the need to go to the emergency room by making sure your baby is taking the proper type and amount of liquids.*
- *Do not offer your baby any medications for vomiting (such as Imodium); these do not work for children.*
- *Notify your doctor if there is blood in the vomit, she has fever for more than seventy-two hours, or has fewer than three wet diapers in a twenty-four-hour period.*

Daddy vs. Doctor—It Bothered Me More Than It Bothered Her

Thankfully, Aubrey remained healthy for the first nine months of her life. Go breast milk! Then, when she was nine months old, she got her first cold. She had a runny nose and a cough and a few days of fever, but overall she was in good spirits.

We thought she was getting better until one morning she vomited. The first time it happened, we assumed she had probably gagged on her mucus and it had caused her to throw up, but an hour later she vomited again. Then again a half hour later. We kept count: she threw up eleven times that day. The funny thing was that it didn't bother her. My wife and I nicknamed her "Puke and Giggle." She would be playing on the floor, her face would suddenly frown, she'd throw up, then she'd point at the puddle in front of her, look up at us, clap and giggle, and go back to playing.

199

It was amazing how resilient she was. I wish I could say the same thing for myself. That night I woke up at two a.m. with horrible stomach cramps and found myself on the floor of the bathroom vomiting and calling for my wife to help. I think I told her I felt like I was going to die.

I have to admit I am not a good patient, and all I could think of was that my nine-month-old handled being sick much better than I did.

Common Sense Facts: Vomiting

Vomiting is usually caused by a viral infection and may last one to two weeks. Vomiting may be present alone or with a combination of symptoms that include diarrhea, fever, and fussiness. Treatment should be focused on supportive care and adequate hydration.

Breastfed infants
- Do not offer any solids or liquids for at least thirty to sixty minutes after vomiting.
- Provide breast milk in smaller amounts (shorter feedings) and more frequently than usual.

Formula-fed infants
- Do not offer any solids or liquids for at least thirty to sixty minutes after vomiting.
- Offer oral rehydration solutions (Pedialyte) or other clear liquids such as sugar water or tea.
- Offer small amounts frequently, gradually increasing the volume. For example, 1 teaspoon, then a couple minutes later another teaspoon, then a couple minutes later 2 teaspoons, and so on.
- If your child vomits while you are increasing the volume, wait another thirty to sixty minutes and start again.
- After four hours of no vomiting, you may return to formula.
- Avoid plain water. (Your body needs electrolytes; water may cause more vomiting.)

If she is at the stage where she is eating solids
- Do not worry if she does not want to eat anything.
- She may lose weight—this is normal, and she will gain it back when she is feeling better.
- Adequate hydration is the most important issue.

Common mistakes in the treatment of vomiting
- Giving liquids or solids too soon (especially water).
- Allowing your child to drink as much as she wants after vomiting instead of starting with small amounts and gradually increasing the volume.
- Using over-the-counter medication.

Call your doctor if
- your baby does not urinate at least three times in a twenty-four-hour period.
- there is blood in the vomit.
- your baby has a fever for more than seventy-two hours.
- your baby is inconsolable.

Hoof and Mouth?—Hand, Foot, and Mouth

Hand, foot, and mouth (HFM)—or as my patients like to refer to it, "hand, hoof, and mouth"—is an infection often seen in the first year of life. For some unknown reason child care facilities freak out about this infection, although it is no more serious than any standard viral infection we see in kids. Hand, foot, and mouth is caused by the *cocksackie* virus and symptoms usually include mouth sores and a rash on the baby's hands and feet. Not every child will have all three symptoms.

Mouth sores, which are red and generally appear on the back of the throat and sides of the mouth or gums are of the greatest concern. They are very painful. If you've ever had a canker sore, imagine ten of them on the back of your throat. Ouch! On top of that, there is no good remedy to relieve the pain. Medications such as Orajel, Chloraseptic spray, or even Tylenol and Motrin

201

offer either fleeting relief or no relief at all. The sores are so painful that your child may not want to eat or drink. She may also drool more than usual because she doesn't want to swallow her own saliva.

HFM may also be accompanied by a rash, which usually appears on the hands and feet, especially the palms and soles. The rash can appear anywhere on the body, including the bottom and groin, but the hands and feet are the most common location. The rash looks like small, fluid-filled pimples on a red base. There may be only a few scattered around or larger groups. The rash is not painful, nor does it scar. And it's not contagious, so don't worry if you touch it.

Your baby may also have a high fever that comes and goes for about seventy-two hours.

Again this is a virus, so antibiotics are inappropriate. Here's how you can treat your child's HFM:

- Give Tylenol or Motrin for fever and pain.
- Most important, make sure your child gets enough fluids. The number one reason children go to the hospital for HFM is dehydration, because they don't want to drink due to the painful mouth sores. Try cool or warm drinks, both of which may feel soothing.
- If she is old enough, you can offer Popsicles, which may feel soothing on the mouth sores and supply about four ounces of liquid.
- Don't worry if your baby doesn't want to eat anything. Her appetite will return once she's feeling better.

Common Sense Bottom Line
The mouth sores may be very painful, but HFM is no more serious than the common cold. Make sure your child has sufficient liquids. After three or four days, the sores will begin healing, the fever will go away, and most children will begin to feel better. The rash may take at least a week to go away.

The "Slapped Cheek" Virus—Fifth's Disease

Another virus seen in children can cause common cold symptoms and fever, but the hallmark is a rash that looks like someone slapped your child's cheeks and a flat, lacy red rash all over her body that blanches (lightens) when you press on it. The rash is not contagious nor does it hurt or itch. Neither the rash nor the cold symptoms is any more dangerous to your child than any other common virus. However, this virus can be dangerous to pregnant women, so if a child at day care gets it, they will notify you and other parents. In pregnant women, it may cause severe anemia to the newborn. Because fifth's disease is caused by a virus there is no treatment other than supportive care until it runs its course.

If you are pregnant and have been exposed to a child with this virus, stay calm; most likely nothing will come of it. But do notify your obstetrician. He or she will check your blood to see if you have antibodies to this infection. Many women have already been exposed to this virus and have built up antibodies, so there is nothing to worry about. If you are not immune, your doctor may monitor you and the fetus more closely.

Common Sense Bottom Line
Slapped cheek is not serious in children. Notify your obstetrician if you are pregnant and exposed to fifth's disease.

Roseola

No more serious than other viral infections, roseola has very specific symptoms: a fever for two to three days, then, twelve to twenty-four hours after the fever breaks, the child breaks out in a rash. The fever may be very high (103 to 105) for those first few days, but this is nothing to worry about. Just treat the fever with Tylenol or Motrin to make your child feel better. The rash looks like tiny red dots that may be flat or raised and may cover your baby from head to toe, although they are most common on the torso. The good news is that the rash doesn't itch or scar or hurt. Don't be surprised, though, if your child remains very fussy for a day or two after the fever goes away, as this is one of the characteristics of roseola. Also, she may or may not have other coldlike symptoms, such as a runny nose and cough.

Even though the rash may look mean, its appearance is a good sign. First of all, it means the fever is gone for good; second, it indicates that your baby is no longer contagious; and finally, we can now identify it as roseola and be assured that your child is going to start feeling better soon. Although the rash may take at least a week to go away, as it doesn't itch or hurt there is no need to put anything on it. Ointments or other preparations will not make it go away any faster.

Common Sense Bottom Line

If your child has a fever for a few days, then gets a rash when the fever breaks, the mystery is solved: she has roseola, which is not serious.

Spots, Dots, and Stripes—Rashes

Babies tend to develop more spots and dots than a zoo animal. There are many different kinds of rashes in children, and though they may look menacing, most are not dangerous. In general, no matter what the rash looks like, if it doesn't bother your child and she seems happy and healthy, there is usually no cause for concern. What you want to know is if the rash needs to be treated, and if so how to do it. Here are some quick tips to help you connect the dots. Rashes can be grouped into three categories:

* Allergic rashes
* Irritant rashes
* Rashes caused by infection (usually viral infections)

You can tell which group your child's rash belongs in by the way the rash looks, its location, and any related symptoms. If the rash is spread all over your child's body, it is usually due to either an allergy or an infection. An allergic rash usually itches, while a rash from an infection, such as a virus, will appear during or shortly after your child has had other cold symptoms. If the rash is located on only one part of the body, it is usually from an irritant that came into contact with that part of the body (like diaper rash).

Let's go through some of the most common rashes your baby might get. I have included Rash Diagnosis and Treatment diagrams (see pages 210–13) to help you figure out what kind of rash your child has and whether or not treatment or a trip to your doctor is necessary.

Hives

One of the most common allergic rashes is hives. Hives are big red blotches that are slightly raised and may have a lighter-colored or white center. One of the characteristics of hives is that the blotches appear and disappear on different parts of the body. For instance, you may notice them all over your child's back and chest, then an hour later those blotches are gone but other blotches have appeared on her face and legs. When many hives are clumped close together, that part of the body may look swollen. This is especially common on the hands and feet. Don't worry: this is a common rash and is not dangerous.

Hives are an allergic reaction to something your child ate, touched, or breathed; they may also accompany a viral infection. Some children break out in hives when they are sick because their body is having an "allergic reaction" to the virus.

Hives can come and go for up to seven to ten days, even after whatever triggered them has been removed. This can make it difficult to pinpoint the cause, unless you noticed that the hives began after a certain trigger.

Here's how you can treat hives:

- Give your baby Children's Benadryl. Benadryl helps blunt the body's allergic reaction and helps alleviate symptoms such as itching. A dosing chart is available on page 266.
- Dress your baby in loose, cool clothing as hives are exacerbated by heat and tight-fitting clothes (which is why hives are often found along the waistband).

205

- Avoid warm baths as these tend to increase the hives. (Cool baths are fine.)
- Don't use anti-inflammatory or anti-itch creams, such as a steroid or Benadryl cream. These have no benefit because the hives are an internal body reaction that manifests on the skin; the skin itself is not the problem.

Common Sense Bottom Line

Hives are no reason to panic. They nearly always seem to go away as quickly as they showed. However, if they are associated with facial swelling or problems breathing, notify your doctor immediately.

Diaper Rash

Diaper rash is the most common rash in infants. There are two main causes of diaper rash:

1. Irritation of the skin from a wet or dirty diaper
2. A secondary yeast infection

Although pesky, neither of these rashes is serious.

A wet diaper can irritate the baby's skin and cause chafing and redness. If this is the case, your child may scream when you try to change her diaper. Even if you are the parent of the year and never let your child sit for an extended period of time in a dirty diaper, your baby will probably still get this rash. To treat this type of diaper rash, known as *diaper dermatitis,* do the following:

- Place a thick barrier of diaper rash cream on the red area every diaper change. The idea is to create a barrier so the skin can heal without getting re-irritated by subsequent wet diapers. You can use any of the products created for this purpose, including Desitin, Balmex, Butt Paste, and Aquaphor. Or you can create your own home remedy using cornstarch and Maalox.

206 • Let your baby go bottomless so that the affected area can get some air. This is beneficial but logistically difficult with a baby who may poop or pee at any moment. So do this at your own risk!

- If the area is very inflamed, use 1 percent cortisone cream twice a day and diaper creams the rest of the time. Over-the-counter steroid creams such as 1 percent hydrocortisone cream are safe for all ages.
- If there are areas of skin that are particularly chafed and raw, use a layer of Neosporin on them first to help prevent a secondary infection, then the diaper cream on top.

Diaper rash may take more than a week to get better and comes and goes as long as your baby is in diapers.

The second type of diaper rash is caused by a *yeast infection*. If your child's diaper rash is not getting better, if the redness is in the creases of the skin, or you see little red bumps around the rash, your baby may have a secondary yeast infection. Also, if you've been using cornstarch to treat the diaper rash and the rash is getting worse, your child's rash is likely a yeast infection that is growing because cornstarch is a food for yeast. Both boys and girls can get a yeast infection at this age because yeast grows in any wet environment, and the diaper area is the perfect setting.

To treat a yeast infection of the diaper area, follow this treatment:

- Use an over-the-counter antiyeast cream, such as Lotrimin, at least three times a day. It is the same cream you would buy for your own athlete's foot and it is safe for newborns. Apply it over the red areas and you should see an improvement in about a week.
- If the rash does not improve after a week, notify your doctor. There are safe prescription antifungal creams such as Nystatin that he or she may want to prescribe.

Dry Skin

You may hear the terms "dry skin," "atopic dermatitis," or "eczema." Don't worry about the semantics. The key here is that the treatment options are basically the same no matter what you call it. Dry skin in infants may be from a family history, allergies, dry weather, or the fact that babies in general have sensitive skin. Whatever the reason, infants commonly need to be treated for dry skin. Fortunately, most outgrow this condition.

Dry skin on your infant may appear in many different ways. Her whole body or parts of her body may feel like sandpaper, with very small, fine skin-colored bumps. If her skin is very dry, there may also be inflammation, with dry, bumpy red areas. This is especially common in the creases of her arms, behind her knees, on her ankles and wrists, and on her cheeks.

If your baby's skin feels dry but you don't see any red bumps, then moisturizer cream is all she needs. There are many different moisturizers on the market, including Eucerin Cream, Aquaphor, Johnson's Baby Cream, and Vaseline petroleum jelly. Each has a different consistency, but they all do the same thing. Choose one that doesn't have extra fragrances or additives that might irritate a baby's sensitive skin and apply it all over your baby's body and face at least three times a day, but as many times as you think about it. This is especially important after bathing because water dries out the skin.

If her skin is dry and there are red patches or bumps, a steroid cream may be needed to decrease the inflammation and help her skin heal more quickly. An over-the-counter steroid cream such as 1 percent cortisone cream is safe and can be used on newborns. I recommend using the steroid cream twice a day for at least one week. If it is helping, keep using it until the rash goes away, and continue using moisturizer as often as possible.

If you don't notice an improvement after one week on the steroid cream, notify your doctor. A stronger prescription cream may be needed.

Cradle Cap

This not-so-attractive skin condition may look intimidating, but it's very common and can be treated easily. It generally appears in the first few months of life but it can occur anytime in the first year. Areas of the scalp, as well as the creases behind the ears, may have thick yellow crusty skin and sometimes areas of redness. The condition may be itchy and irritating to your baby.

Since this is a type of dry skin, some of the same treatments can be utilized. When the rash is behind the ears, use moisturizer cream and cortisone cream. The moisturizer helps the dryness, and the cortisone cream treats the redness. If the rash affects the scalp, you'll want to use either baby oil or a special shampoo (such as Selsun Blue or Neutrogena T/Gel) to soften up the crust and gently rub it away. Massage the shampoo or oil into your baby's hair and scalp and leave it on for about five minutes. Then wash it out with a soft brush or washcloth, making sure that you cover and protect your baby's eyes. It may take several applications, but this should do the trick.

Rashes Caused by Viral Infections

Many different viruses can cause a rash. Some are serious, but most are harmless. Since a number of viral rashes are similar in appearance, the best way to tell if a rash indicates a serious condition is to observe how your child looks and behaves. If she has a rash but is acting fairly normal (take into consideration that she's sick with a virus), her condition probably isn't serious.

In general, viral rashes consist of small red dots that are flat in some areas and bumpy in others. Viral rashes may cover your child from head to toe, but they're most common on the torso. Such rashes usually don't itch or bother your child, and they may appear during or shortly after other viral symptoms, such as congestion, runny nose, cough, and fever. A viral rash usually consists of red dots that blanch (lighten) when you press on them, and the rash usually resolves on its own within a week.

If your child's rash does not blanch, you should notify your doctor immediately. This may be a sign of a more serious infection. One such rash, called *petechia,* looks like the skin was dotted with a red felt-tip pen. If this rash is associated with a serious illness, your child will also appear very ill, as is the case with meningitis.

You may also see this type of rash on the chest or face after a child coughs or vomits violently. This is absolutely normal and no cause for alarm, but notify your doctor if the rash is spreading or you are concerned.

If your child has a rash that is comprised of clear fluid-filled **209** bumps (vesicles), she should also be seen by her doctor. One example of this type of rash is chicken pox.

Common Sense Bottom Line

If your baby looks basically fine and is not bothered by the rash, don't worry about it.

If the rash does not blanch or there are clear, fluid-filled bumps, or your child appears very ill, notify your physician.

Rash Localized to Diaper Area
Diagnosis and Treatment

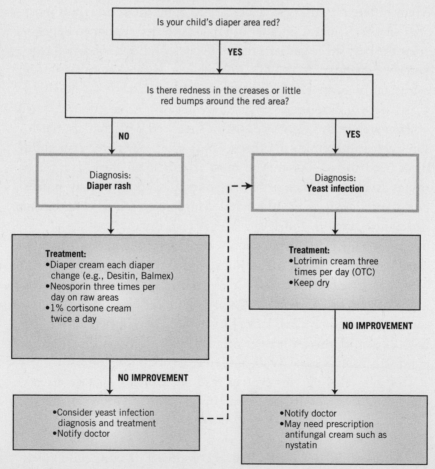

Is your child's diaper area red?

YES

Is there redness in the creases or little red bumps around the red area?

NO   YES

Diagnosis: **Diaper rash**

Diagnosis: **Yeast infection**

Treatment:
• Diaper cream each diaper change (e.g., Desitin, Balmex)
• Neosporin three times per day on raw areas
• 1% cortisone cream twice a day

Treatment:
• Lotrimin cream three times per day (OTC)
• Keep dry

NO IMPROVEMENT

NO IMPROVEMENT

• Consider yeast infection diagnosis and treatment
• Notify doctor

• Notify doctor
• May need prescription antifungal cream such as nystatin

210

Rash Localized to Creases/Skin Folds Diagnosis and Treatment

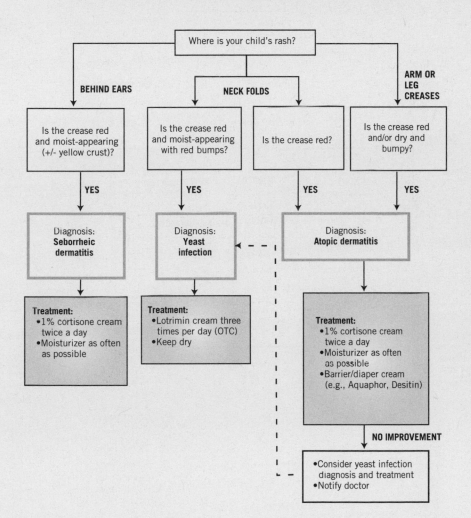

Rash Localized to Scalp Diagnosis and Treatment

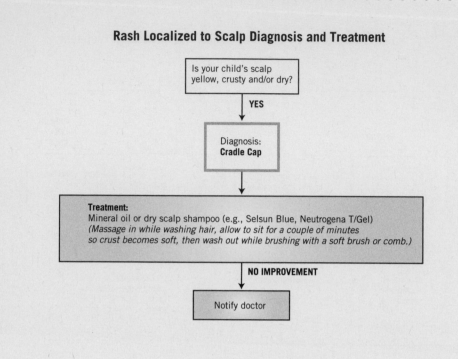

Generalized Rash Diagnosis and Treatment

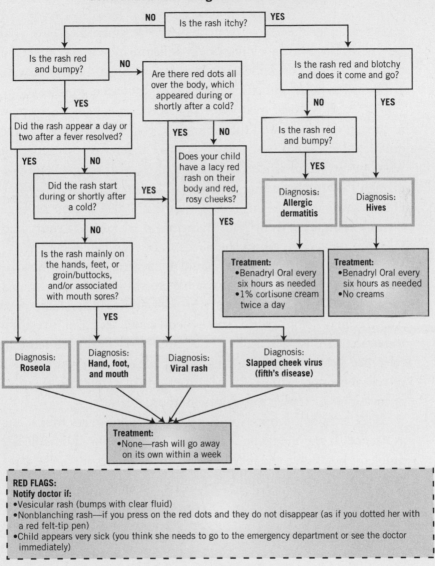

RED FLAGS:
Notify doctor if:
- Vesicular rash (bumps with clear fluid)
- Nonblanching rash—if you press on the red dots and they do not disappear (as if you dotted her with a red felt-tip pen)
- Child appears very sick (you think she needs to go to the emergency department or see the doctor immediately)

Whistle While You Work—Wheezing

Children under the age of two often wheeze when they have viral infections. That's because viruses cause inflammation in the airways of the lungs, which causes the airways to narrow. Since a baby's airways are narrow to begin with, further narrowing causes her to wheeze.

Although we may treat wheezing in the same way as we treat asthma, it does not mean that your child has asthma. In fact, some children don't need to be treated at all. We refer to this group of wheezers as "happy wheezers," because their wheezing isn't intense enough to cause breathing problems. On the other hand, in some children who are wheezing, you'll see the muscles in their rib cage or neck being used to help force air into their lungs. If your child falls into the second group, she needs to be seen by her doctor.

The doctor will listen to your child's lungs and watch her breathing to determine if she is having trouble breathing. If it is determined that she is working hard to breathe, a medication called Albuterol or Xopenex may be prescribed. These medications are administered in the form of a mist, which she can breathe easily through a mask in the office. I call it "breathing the clouds." The medicine immediately relaxes the smooth muscle around her airways, allowing them to open so that air travels through them more freely.

If the medicine works, you can use it at home every four hours as needed. If the medicine does not work and your child still has problems breathing, she may need further medication, such as steroids, or further testing and treatment in the hospital.

Snap, Crackle, and Pop—Bronchiolitis

Some children contract an illness called *bronchiolitis*. A child with bronchiolitis will have normal cold symptoms such as fever, cough, and congestion; however, the virus also causes inflammation in the smallest airways of the lungs called *bronchioles* (in contrast to bronchitis, which is an infection of larger airways of the lungs). When you listen to a child with bronchiolitis it sounds as if they have Rice Krispies in their lungs because their breathing is crackly and wheezy. Depending on the amount of lung involvement, the child may have trouble breathing.

If a child with bronchiolitis sounds crackly and wheezy but is not having problems breathing, then just watch and wait. Because bronchiolitis is caused by a virus, antibiotics will not help your child get better. The recommended treatment for bronciolitis is to:

- Use a vaporizer.
- Make sure your child has adequate fluids.
- Make sure your child has adequate rest.
- If your child is having trouble breathing, she may be treated with Albuterol to open up the lungs and make it easier for her to breathe. Although studies have not shown an overall benefit with this medication, clinically some children do show improvement.

The only reason to admit a child with bronchiolitis to the hospital is if her breathing worsens and she needs oxygen and supplemental fluids. This is more common in premature infants. Fortunately, most children with bronchiolitis are "happy wheezers" and never get to this point.

See No Evil, Hear No Evil—Eye and Ear Concerns

Eyes and ears can be the source of discomfort for little ones. During the first year of life, babies seem to be constantly tugging at their ears or being sent home from day care because of red eyes or discharge. As discussed, sometimes the fact that she's pulling on her ears has nothing to do with pain. She may just be exploring this fascinating part of her body. If she does have a problem with her ears or her eyes, however, most of the time it's nothing serious and can be treated easily.

Ear Infections
A child may pull on her ears for a number of reasons other than an infection. Your child may feel referred pain from an erupting tooth or from pressure caused by nasal congestion. Or she may have an

215

inner or outer ear infection. So how can you tell if she has an ear infection?

First of all, there are two types of ear infections: *inner ear infections* and *outer ear infections*. Inner ear infections are the most common and are caused by fluid in the middle ear when a child has a cold.

If your child is pulling her ears and has other cold symptoms, such as fever, cough, or congestion, she either has an *inner ear infection* or feels pressure in her ears from nasal congestion. A doctor should examine her to see whether or not she has an ear infection. If she does, you'll have several treatment options. Since an ear infection can be caused by a virus or bacteria, and viral infections go away on their own, not all ear infections need to be treated with antibiotics. The latest thinking in pediatrics is that it's best to wait forty-eight hours before treating some infections, to see if they will go away on their own.

If your child has ear pain, a fever, and has been up all night, and if your doctor sees an ear infection, I would recommend starting antibiotics because your baby will likely feel better by the following morning. If, on the other hand, your baby has a cold but doesn't seem to have ear pain, and your doctor happens to see an ear infection, I would suggest giving you a prescription for antibiotics and telling you to hold on to it. If your child starts to have a fever or you notice that her ear hurts, then you would start the medication.

Outer ear infections are caused by getting water in the ear, and they can be very painful, especially when you pull on the outside of the ear. If your child has an outer ear infection, you may notice a yellow discharge from the ear due to the inflammation of the outer ear canal. Outer ear infections can be treated easily with antibiotic ear drops, which your doctor will prescribe.

Just because your baby gets water in her ear doesn't mean she'll get an outer ear infection. Do take precautions, however, by drying her ears as best you can *with a towel* after her bath or when she goes in the pool. *Don't use anything like a Q-tip because you may cause irritation or damage the eardrum or outer ear canal.*

Ear Pain That Isn't Caused by an Ear Infection
A baby may pull on her ears when she's teething or if she has sores in her mouth from a virus such as hand, foot, and mouth. Since a

child of this age may not be able to pinpoint where the pain is coming from, she may pull on her left ear if a molar is coming in on the left side. Or she might pull on her right ear if she has a sore on the right side of her mouth. Investigate to get to the source of her pain.

The problem may be with the skin behind her ears, so be sure to check there, too. This is a common area where children develop dry, cracked skin, which can be itchy and irritating. (See page 207 for dry skin treatment options.)

Ear Complaint Diagnosis and Treatment

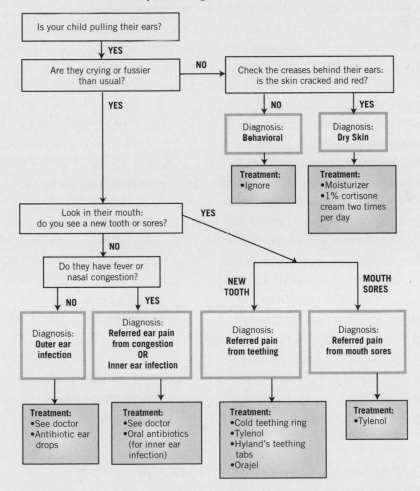

Red Eyes or Discharge from the Eyes

Discharge may be caused by a clogged tear duct, infection, or even overflow from the nose. If the eye has discharge but it's not red, the discharge is usually caused by a clogged tear duct or overflow from the nose. If the eye has discharge and is red, the discharge is usually an infection or allergy. Each of these conditions is easily treated and rarely serious.

Clogged Tear Duct

Healthy newborns often have yellow discharge from their eyes. If you see this but the white of the eye remains white, it is usually a clogged tear duct. Tear ducts run from the corner of your eyes closest to the nose down the side of the nose. The tear duct connects the eye to the nose and that is why when you cry you get a runny nose. In infants, the tear duct is very small and sometimes gets blocked. If your baby has a mildly blocked tear duct, she will have a teary eye with clear discharge. If the duct is *very* clogged, she will have a thick yellow discharge. Neither case is serious. The discharge will be most noticeable when your child wakes up and her eyelids are glued shut. You will be able to tell that this is not an infection because the white of the eye will remain white, unlike conjunctivitis, or "pink" eye. You may notice, however, that the rim of her upper or lower eyelid does look a little red because the discharge is irritating, and the lid is further irritated when you wipe the discharge from her eye.

Treat a clogged tear duct by doing the following:

- Gently massage her tear duct up and down with your pinky finger to help push discharge into the nose and eye and bypass the obstruction.
- If you are breastfeeding, place a few drops of breast milk in the corner of her eye to help lubricate the duct and prevent infection.
- Use a warm compress to gently remove any discharge and help to clean the eye.

A clogged tear duct may come and go for up to one year and usually resolves permanently by that time. It may be in only one eye, both eyes, or alternate between the two. Notify your pediatrician if

the discharge persists after one year of age or is accompanied by redness of the white of the eye. If the tear duct remains clogged after a
year, referral to an ophthalmologist is warranted because the duct may
need to be probed or a small stent may need to be inserted to hold the
duct open. This is a quick outpatient procedure.

Overflow from the Nose

If your child has yellow discharge from her eyes, and the white
of her eye remains white, but she also has nasal congestion, she
may have overflow from the nose. Since the nose and eyes are connected, any time there is mucus in the nose it may leak into the
eyes. Again, this is usually most noticeable when your child wakes
up from sleeping and may cause her eyes to be glued shut. There
is no treatment for this type of discharge except wiping the mucus
out of the eye and waiting until the congestion goes away.

Infection or Allergy

If your child has a red eye, it is usually due to an infection or an allergy.

- If the white of the eye is red, itchy, and watery, it is usually
  due to an allergy called *allergic conjunctivitis*. This can be
  treated with a prescription allergy eye drop.
- If the white of the eye is red with watery discharge, not
  itchy, it is usually *viral conjunctivitis*, or *pink eye*. The infant
  may or may not have other coldlike symptoms. Since this
  type of conjunctivitis is due to a virus, there is no specific
  treatment other than time.
- If the white of the eye is red and there is yellow discharge,
  your child may have *bacterial conjunctivitis* and benefit
  from antibiotic eyedrops.

In general, conjunctivitis, whether bacterial or viral, is very contagious. Make sure to keep your child's hands out of her eyes (and your
eyes) as much as possible and wash her hands immediately if she rubs
her eyes "by accident." Rubbing the eyes is also a good way for viral
conjunctivitis to turn into a bacterial conjunctivitis, because bacteria
from the hands are introduced into the eyes. When your child has

219

conjunctivitis it is a good idea for her to use different towels and to make sure not to share bedding or pillows with other family members.

Common Sense Bottom Line

Eye infections are generally not serious, nor are they a cause for concern. If the eye does not improve with the proper treatment, looks swollen all the way around the eye, or is popping out (not common) notify your doctor.

Eye Complaint Diagnosis and Treatment

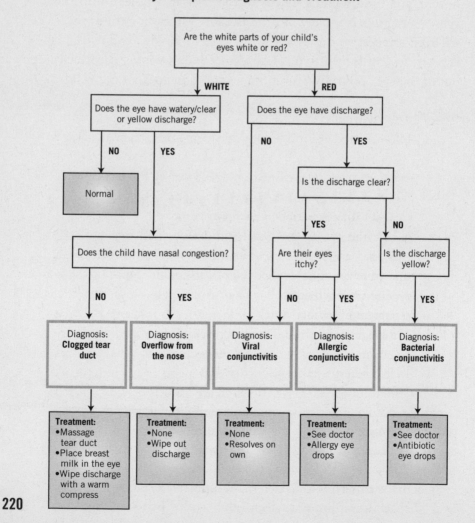

CHAPTER 10

PROTECT

Vaccines

. . . .

*"For those who believe, no proof is necessary. For those who
don't believe, no proof is possible."*
                                    —Stuart Chase, writer and economist

The purpose of this chapter is to focus on the so-called vaccine
debate. While medical professionals, and most parents, agree
that vaccines are an important component of a child's health,
recent concerns over the possible risks of vaccines have overshad-
owed their enormous benefits.

Today's parents are flooded with information on vaccines—some
of it is valuable, but much of it (though well-intentioned) is incor-
rect. With so much information out there on the Internet and in
the media, it is often hard to tell which statements concerning vaccines are based on scientific truth, which are based on emotion, and
which are simply fabricated out of thin air. So, who can you trust?

When I meet with parents, I continue to hear these three concerns about vaccinating their baby:

1. Some vaccines, specifically the measles, mumps, rubella
   (MMR) vaccine, may cause autism.

221

2. Certain components of vaccines, such as mercury and aluminum, may cause autistic symptoms or developmental delay.
3. We give so many vaccines nowadays that we are overloading
a baby's immune system.

In this chapter, I want to explain and demystify each of these
concerns:

- Vaccines and autism
- Vaccines and mercury and aluminum
- Vaccines and "overloading" a baby's immune system

Vaccines and Autism

The vaccine for measles, mumps, and rubella (MMR) has been
accused of causing autism. The "debate" started over two ideas.

*1. A relationship was noted between the timing of the MMR vac-
cine and the diagnosis of autism.*

The MMR vaccine is given at one year of age and autism is usually diagnosed between eighteen and twenty-four months of age. As
a result, based on this temporal correlation, a hypothesis was formed
that questioned whether the MMR vaccine *caused* autism. It seemed
a telling coincidence. If you put something into the body (in this
case the MMR vaccine) and shortly thereafter something develops
(in this case autism), maybe that first thing caused the second thing.
Unfortunately, what grabs the headlines and what sticks in people's
minds is the *hypothesis* rather than the studies attempting to sub-
stantiate it. Several studies have looked at a possible link between
the MMR vaccine and autism and have failed to find one. One
such study in the United Kingdom that evaluated nearly five hundred autistic children showed no change in the rate of autism after
the MMR vaccine was introduced in 1987. There was no increase
in diagnoses around the time children received the MMR vaccine
and there were no differences in the rate of autism between the vac-

cinated and unvaccinated groups. Several other studies around the world, including the United States, Canada, Finland, and Denmark, looking at thousands of children have shown similar results. The fact is that the studies which looked into a possible link between the MMR and autism found there was no link.

Common Sense Bottom Line

Reputable scientific studies that looked into a possible link between the MMR vaccine and autism concluded there was no link.

2. A study published by Dr. Andrew Wakefield in 1998 made reference to a possible link between autism and the MMR vaccine.

Believe it or not, this one study was the basis for just about everything we now hear about a possible link between vaccines and autism. Dr. Wakefield's study was based on suggested findings in *twelve children*. That's right. Despite multiple studies showing no link between the MMR vaccine and autism, and the fact that not one study has been able to duplicate Dr. Wakefield's results nor show a link between any vaccine (including the MMR) and autism, his study, based on only twelve children, has led thousands of parents to question the advisability of the MMR vaccine.

Unfortunately, Dr. Wakefield's article was so influential that families began to defer vaccinating their children against measles, mumps, and rubella. As a result, there has been a rise in these infections and deaths because of these diseases since the article was published more than a decade ago.

News of the alleged connection between the MMR vaccine and autism has flooded the media ever since Wakefield's study was published. Newspapers, mainstream magazines, and popular talk shows have covered the issue, and celebrities have lent their opinions to the debate. Now you might ask, "But isn't one study enough?" If the study was a scientifically sound one, you would have a good point. Despite all the media attention given to this debate, few people have heard that Dr. Wakefield's study (the only study suggesting a link) *has been thoroughly discredited.* In 2004, ten of thirteen researchers involved in this study came out with a statement saying, "We wish to make clear that in this paper no causal link was established between the MMR vaccine and autism as the data was insufficient." This statement was made when evidence came to light about how Dr. Wakefield performed and helped to fund his study.

In fact, a portion of Dr. Wakefield's study was funded by a law firm representing families suing vaccine companies over the possible adverse effects of the vaccines that their children received. Several of the children in Dr. Wakefield's study were represented by the law firm suing the vaccine companies. Not only is this an obvious conflict of interest, but Dr. Wakefield was also found to have manipulated data and was shown to display questionable ethics. For example, he paid the children in his study five pounds (he's from England) to draw their blood at his son's birthday party.

Although it was not directly in response to Wakefield's study, in February 2009, a special U.S. federal court ruled that there is no link between the MMR vaccine and autism. Special Master Denise Vowell said that the evidence "is weak, contradictory, and unpersuasive . . . sadly, the petitioners in this litigation have been the victims of bad science conducted to support litigation rather than to advance medical and scientific understanding."

Unfortunately, we don't yet know what causes autism. And although it would be easy to blame vaccines, we cannot create a false cause simply because we haven't yet found the real one. Since there has been no link established between vaccines and autism, blaming vaccinations is no different from blaming a myriad of other unknown factors, including increased environmental pollutants, the shrinking ozone, increased cell phone usage, the increase in power lines, the increase in maternal age of first-time parents, and psychological stressors during pregnancy. My point is not to individually blame any specific trigger but merely point out that we do not know the trigger as of yet, and vaccines, on which we have focused most of our attention, have yielded no correlation.

The key here is that we should continue investigating all possible causes of autism. And we shouldn't conclude that vaccines are the cause without any evidence to support that claim. Autism has a significant genetic component (as noted in research comparing autism in identical twins versus fraternal twins), and there has been the discovery of several genes that have been linked to autism. In May 2009, researchers at the University of California, Los Angeles (UCLA), announced the discovery of the autism-risk gene on chromosome 17, which may explain the disparity in autism rates between boys and girls (boys are four times more likely to have autism compared to girls). And there are probably environmental triggers that cause autism to manifest. I do not believe we will find an individual factor that, if eliminated, will eradicate autism. On the other hand, we may be able to limit autism by avoiding certain environmental triggers in susceptible individuals. At the time of this book's publication, we do not know what those triggers are.

Common Sense Bottom Line
Reputable scientific studies have shown that there is no evidence proving that vaccines cause autism.

Vaccines and Mercury and Aluminum

Another reason many parents are concerned about vaccines is the chemicals or preservatives in them. Many people believe that these components may cause autism or autistic-like symptoms. The two most commonly sighted components are thimerosal and aluminum.

Thimerosal
Thimerosal is a mercury-like compound that was often used as a preservative in vaccines in order to keep them from becoming contaminated by germs. Because of adverse effects to the central nervous system (CNS) of individuals exposed to high doses of mercury, another well-meaning hypothesis was created: if high doses of mercury may affect the CNS, and we use a form of mercury in vaccines, maybe this form (thimerosal) causes problems as well. Although the signs and symptoms of mercury poisoning have

been equated to autism, they are, in fact, distinctly different. This means that the link between thimerosal and autism is implausible to begin with. Still, a possible link was studied

Once again the studies were unable to link thimerosal with autism. First of all, although thimerosal is similar to mercury, it is actually a different compound and doesn't cause the same side effects as high doses of mercury. Second, if you added up all the thimerosal you received in a lifetime and put it into one shot, the amount you received would be so minuscule it could not be proven to have any negative effect.

Even though no link was found between thimerosal and autism, as of 2001 thimerosal was no longer added to vaccines because it was deemed to be an unnecessary preservative. (The only vaccine that still has thimerosal is the multidose flu vaccine given to adults and children over three years of age.) Interestingly, in the years since thimerosal was removed from the vaccines, autism rates have continued to rise. This finding alone shows that thimerosal is not the cause of autism.

Aluminum

Aluminum is used as an *adjuvant* in vaccines, meaning it helps the vaccine create a better immune response. Without an adjuvant, such as aluminum, your child would need more doses of the vaccine to provide adequate protection against infection. Aluminum has been used safely in vaccines for more than seventy-five years. However, because of impaired neurologic development seen with high doses of aluminum, another hypothetical link was created between aluminum and autism.

I agree with experts who have suggested that more studies of aluminum in vaccines must be conducted; however, I do not agree with the alarm that has been raised about aluminum and the warnings that have been made to families. Nor do I think it is necessary to separate required vaccines or use an alternative schedule when administering them.

Here's why:

Aluminum is a naturally occurring element in the earth's crust. It is in our water, food, the air we breathe, and even in breast milk. An infant receives significantly more aluminum in the first six months of life through breast milk or formula than vaccines (about 4.4 milligrams of aluminum from vaccines, 7 milligrams from breast milk, 38 milligrams from formula, and 117 milligrams from soy formula). This fact is conveniently left out of most antivaccine literature. If you plan on not vaccinating your baby because of concerns over aluminum exposure, you might as well stop breastfeeding for the same reason. And if you think formula is a better option, it's not. There is more aluminum in formula than in breast milk. Of course, I don't want you to stop breastfeeding or feeding your infant formula; I just want to put the facts in perspective.

Unfortunately, what is happening with the vaccine debate is that people have isolated certain ingredients that are included in very small quantities in childhood vaccines and concluded that "If high doses of X cause a problem, then small doses must as well." This is a big leap and usually not a correct one. The most potent chemicals, if diluted enough, will not cause harm. For example, I live in Los Angeles. As with the air in most major cities, one breath of Los Angeles air contains pesticides, arsenic, PCPs, tobacco smoke, mold, and mildew. Each ingredient in high quantities would kill us, but I don't see anyone walking down the street wearing a gas mask or holding his breath.

Unless proven otherwise, trace amounts of a chemical will not do any harm just because large quantities of it do. Our bodies are very efficient at filtering out what we need and excreting what we do not, and aluminum is no exception. Fifty to 75 percent of your daily intake of aluminum is excreted within twenty-four hours if you have normal kidneys, which most of us do. High doses of aluminum were found to be a problem in premature infants on dialysis, meaning their dysfunctional kidneys were unable to get rid of the aluminum, causing it to build up in their system. This is not the case in healthy infants with normal kidney function.

My point is this: it is crucial that you read the information you come across with a very critical eye. I understand being concerned

227

when you hear that "high doses of aluminum cause neurologic problems, and there is aluminum in the vaccines your child may take." But when you find out that "the amount of aluminum is very limited, and excess aluminum is easily excreted by your baby's healthy body," your concerns should be alleviated.

Common Sense Bottom Line
The amount of aluminum in vaccines is safe.

Vaccines and Overloading a Baby's Immune System

Some people contend that because children receive more vaccines today than ever before, their systems are "overloaded." To combat this perceived threat to a child's health, *alternative vaccine schedules* have been proposed. It may seem reasonable that by limiting the number of vaccines injected into a child's body at any one time, you are preventing the possibility of "overloading" the body with too many foreign substances. In actuality, however, vaccines, regardless of how many are injected at the same time, do not "overload" or weaken your child's immune system. In fact, vaccines do the exact opposite: they strengthen the immune system. They do this by introducing *antigens* (foreign substances), which prompt the production of antibodies, which in turn cause an immune response. The burden on your child's immune system is much greater from everyday infections such as the common cold or being exposed to germs on a shared toy.

In the early 1960s, children were given five vaccines: those for diphtheria, tetanus, pertussis (whooping cough), smallpox, and polio. The total number of antigenic proteins in those five vaccines was about 3,217. Today we inoculate children with eleven routine vaccines, but because we do a better job purifying them, the total number of antigens in them is fewer than 130 (95 percent fewer antigens). Yes, children receive more shots today, but in fact, we are protecting them against more illnesses while at the same time introducing far fewer foreign substances into their bodies. So it's a win-win.

Then there is the question of side effects from the shots. If your child receives multiple shots at the same time, she will have one episode of side effects. These may include pain at the injection site, local redness or swelling, or a few days of fever or fussiness. However, if you give the vaccines on separate days, you'll be putting her through multiple painful shot episodes and the chance of having side effects after each individual shot. Why would you want that? In addition to increasing the time that your child is susceptible to very serious infection, you'll be increasing the number of side effects she may experience.

Still, some parents argue that their baby is too young to receive so many shots. "She's so tiny," they tell me, "let's wait a couple of months until her immune system is more mature and she can handle the shots better." Again, this is a false perception. The age at which the first vaccines are given is based on two important factors:

1. We want to protect the child as early as possible, because the younger the child the more serious the infection can be.
2. The child needs to be old enough so that her immune system response is adequately developed, because there is no sense giving the vaccine if it won't boost the child's immunity.

Initial vaccines are given at six to eight weeks of life because at this age your child has an adequate immune system and response to the vaccinations, and because it is early enough to protect her from infections that can be very severe in young infants.

Daddy vs. Doctor—The Vaccine Debate

Before we had our daughter, when parents asked me about vaccines I would quote the medical studies and scientific data and moms and dads appeared satisfied. After Aubrey was born, when I started to explain the same information, parents would interrupt me and ask, "What did you decide to do for your daughter?" After telling them I followed the current recommendations by the American Academy of Pediatrics and vaccinated her, I would often hear parents say, "That's good enough for us." Some families wanted to learn about the science behind the vaccines, while others just wanted to know what I had decided for my own child. Still others quoted celebrity activists, such as Jenny McCarthy, or popular books, such as *The Vaccine Book* by Dr. Robert Sears, and didn't want to listen to any other opinions.

I don't think I truly understood the concern about vaccines until I had my own child. As a doctor, I have always felt and continue to feel that vaccines are safe and extremely effective. I have seen children die of preventable diseases, and as an advocate for children's health I feel it is my responsibility to make sure that my patients get vaccinated against them.

However, as a father, I get it. Despite all the scientific research concluding that vaccines are safe, it is hard not to be emotional about the issue. When I took my daughter for her two-month visit with her pediatrician (the first shot visit), every bad thought flooded my mind. In that moment, I was my baby's dad, not a doctor, and my emotional side initially took over. Everything that every "vaccine-questioning" parent had said ran through my head: *What if the scientific studies have been wrong? What if I do something to hurt her? What if vaccines do cause autism? She is so small and perfect right now, what if I do something to change that?*

After that surge of emotion, my practical side kicked in, and I told myself, *I have seen children die of these illnesses, what if Aubrey was one of them? What if she got one of these horrible diseases and was very sick or died or infected another child? Then how would I feel?* This absolute risk clearly outweighed any theoretical unproven one.

Vaccines Make (Common) Sense!

Vaccines have probably done more to decrease disease and death in the last hundred years than any other technological advancement. Now we rarely see illnesses that once killed hundreds of thousands of people. Because we tend to take vaccinations for granted, we forget that parents used to worry about their child catching measles, mumps, or chicken pox from a playmate. Today, when parents ask me to delay a vaccine such as the MMR, I often respond by asking:

"If you found out that a friend's baby just came down with the measles, what would you do?"

They usually answer, "We would come back and get the vaccine."

And I respond with, "What about your concern over autism?" At this point, the parents realize that they have taken for granted that measles isn't a threat, because children routinely get vaccinated to prevent it.

Unfortunately, measles is making a comeback. During a 2008 measles outbreak in San Diego, several families who had deferred the MMR vaccine when their babies were a year old came back to the office wanting their children immunized immediately. But isn't it foolish to wait to have your child immunized until an outbreak of an utterly preventable disease?

There were more cases of measles in 2008 than any year to date since 1996. Sadly, these infections are popping up in unvaccinated communities with more than 90 percent of those infected having not been vaccinated or having an unknown vaccination status. And because of the unwarranted scare about vaccines causing autism, more than 2.5 percent of parents in the United States choose not to vaccinate their children (a rate that has more than doubled in the last decade). However, there are elementary school districts that report much higher rates of vaccine deferral. A recent survey of California schools found that in some schools more than 50 percent of their kindergarteners had not been vaccinated. All but two states currently allow children to go to school without vaccines if it is "against their family's religion," and twenty states now allow

231

children to go to school without vaccines if it is "against their family's belief"—meaning they just don't want them. As a father, this is a huge concern. It puts my daughter and yours directly at risk. Even though Aubrey is up to date with her vaccinations, because she is only eleven months old she has yet to receive the full dose of vaccines. What if an unvaccinated child exposes her to a harmful disease—a disease that is easily preventable?

In January 2009, an unvaccinated Minnesota baby died of Hib infection (Haemophilus influenzae type B) and four others were infected. One child was five months old and partially vaccinated, one child was fully vaccinated but found to have an immunodeficiency. The other three, including the child who died, were unvaccinated—per their parents' decision.

Prior to the Hib vaccine in 1992, there were more than twenty thousand cases a year of Hib and about a thousand deaths a year. Since the vaccine that incidence has dropped nearly 99 percent.

I know that no matter what I say and no matter what evidence I provide, there are those who are so fixed in their beliefs that they will not change their mind. If you take anything from this chapter, however, please look closely at those from whom you are receiving your vaccine advice. Keep an open mind, and speak with your doctor. You wouldn't go to your accountant for dental advice, would you? There are many well-intentioned people, some with considerable media exposure, whose advice is no more credible than your accountant's guidance on when to get a root canal.

Your doctor's recommendation concerning your baby's vaccinations is not a government conspiracy or a story line from an old *X-Files* episode. Doctors do not have ulterior motives for giving your child her vaccines. They are not receiving kickbacks from the pharmaceutical industry. In fact, many physicians actually lose money on the vaccines they administer because of the rising costs of the vaccines and the declining reimbursement by insurance companies.

Anecdotal evidence is not sufficient to prove a true cause and effect. If it were, we would still believe that the world is flat. Those who are spreading the antivaccine message are doing a great disservice to children and potentially causing great harm. Walk into any children's hospital or speak to a parent who had a child die from an infection that could have been prevented with a vaccine, and consider how you feel about your vaccine decision.

Now that you have been part of this chapter's dialogue and are aware of the facts surrounding this issue, I hope you will conclude, along with me and the rest of the medical establishment, that there is no link between vaccines and autism.

Common Sense Bottom Line

Consider the source when you are evaluating something as important as whether or not to vaccinate your baby against serious diseases. And remember, there is no link between vaccines and autism.

CHAPTER 11

FUN

In the Sun and Elsewhere

• •

Contrary to my book's title, babies like to do more than just eat, sleep, and poop. They like to have fun, too. They like to pull on your long hair, poke square blocks through round holes, and pat the dog's tail. Appreciate the time you spend with your infant during this first year, because the fun will never be quite as goofy or surprising as it is at this age.

There are health and safety issues to be aware of when it comes to a baby's good time, including those relating to fun in the sun. I've seen many a sunburned baby, and I've also seen the tragedy of drowning or near-drowning more times than I'd like to recall. Is it necessary to paint your baby's skin white with zinc oxide to prevent sunburn? And is a baby wearing water wings and a life vest completely safe? What about Fido or Kitty—can they be trusted around your baby?

In this chapter I'll address:

- What to look for in a sunscreen
- The "babies are natural swimmers" theory
- The appropriate age to allow babies to enjoy the water
- What to look for in an insect repellant
- How to treat insect bites and allergic reactions
- Babies, cats, and dogs

- Traveling with your baby
- Should your baby watch TV?

Red as a Beet—Sun Protection

Your baby will love to play outside when the weather permits, and you'll appreciate the chance to get out of the house with her to get some fresh air and maintain your sanity. However, sun exposure and sunburns can be potentially dangerous to your child, so proper sun protection is a must.

All children should wear sunscreen that has at least SPF 30 protection. Most baby sunscreens have an SPF of at least 50, which means that your baby can potentially stay in the sun fifty times longer without getting sunburned than if she were not wearing sunscreen at all. Since your infant has no reason to sport a healthy tan, the higher the SPF the better.

The sunscreen should also protect against both UVA and UVB radiation. UVB radiation causes sunburn, skin cancer, and contributes to aging. For years this was the only wavelength that sunscreens protected against. Now most of them prevent against UVA radiation as well. We have learned that UVA radiation damages the deeper layers of the skin, playing an important role in wrinkles and the development of melanoma. Also, UVA rays are equally prevalent all year round and can penetrate through barriers such as windows.

Since infants tend to have sensitive skin, it is best to choose a sunscreen that does not contain chemical additives or fragrances. One such additive found in many sunscreens is PABA, a chemical used to absorb UVB radiation. PABA can cause skin rashes and allergic reactions, so look for sunscreens that are PABA-free.

Finally, make sure to apply the sunscreen on your child early and often. Sunscreen should be applied twenty to thirty minutes prior to exposure and reapplied throughout the day, especially if your child has been in the water. *Water resistant* sunscreens protect for forty minutes of continuous water exposure compared to eighty minutes of protection with *waterproof* sunscreens. Either way, sunscreen can easily be washed away, so remember to reapply it after your baby gets out of the water.

Many parents ask, "How old does our child need to be before we can apply sunscreen?" It seems they've been told that they should not use sunscreen on infants younger than six months of age. This is not exactly true. I would recommend keeping any infant under two months of age out of direct sunlight, but after that make sure to use the sunscreen as needed. My guess is that the recommendation to hold off on sunscreen until six months old was made to keep parents from basking in the sun with their infants (who would do that anyway?), thereby exposing their infant's delicate skin to the harmful rays of the sun and risking a serious burn. You could also make the argument that because of their sensitive skin, babies have a greater chance of having a reaction to the lotion. In fact, sunscreen is safe and can be used on babies under six months of age. You'll find a number of sunscreens at your local drugstore that are safe and made specifically for babies, including Water BABIES, California Baby, and BullFrog. If you are concerned about a possible reaction, place a small amount on your baby's leg first as a test patch.

Sunscreen should always be used in conjunction with proper clothing, such as a hat and T-shirt, and you should keep your child in the shade at least part of the time you're outdoors.

Common Sense Bottom Line

Keep babies younger than two months old out of direct sunlight. After that, use a baby sunscreen whenever you're in the sun. Choose one with an SPF of at least 30 (preferably 50), and make sure it protects against UVA and UVB and is PABA-free.

Buzz Off—Insect Bites and Stings

Spending time in the great outdoors can be lots of fun, but it can also have its downside. Insect bites and stings, for example, are a concern for parents, especially in the summertime. Most insect bites and stings can be avoided or safely treated without complication. Although there is the possibility that a child may have a severe allergic reaction to a bite, such reactions are rare.

Insects tend to come out more around dusk and dawn and around stagnant pools of water, so if you are taking walks around these times or places be particularly careful. Insect repellant with up to a 30 percent concentration of DEET is safe for children over two months of age, as well as for breastfeeding women. DEET is the active ingredient proven to work in insect repellants. Clothing that covers most of your baby's body can provide excellent protection as well, and should be used in conjunction with the insect repellant. When you apply the repellant, be sure to avoid your child's hands and feet because they usually end up in her mouth. Putting the repellant on her arms and legs is usually sufficient to protect her hands and feet.

If your child does get a bite, don't worry; she'll be fine. The only consequences you'll likely have to deal with are redness, inflammation, and itching. To treat simple itching, oral Benadryl works best. If the area around the bite is very swollen and red, it is usually not an infection but rather an allergic reaction. This can be easily treated with oral Benadryl every six hours as needed. Benadryl will blunt the body's allergic response, decreasing the redness, swelling, and itching. You can also place a small amount of 1 percent cortisone cream on the red area twice a day to decrease the inflammation. If there is a break in the skin, I suggest applying Neosporin a few times a day to help prevent a secondary infection, especially if your child is scratching the bite.

If your child is stung by a bee, it is important to remove the stinger. You can do this by taking your fingernail or the tip of a tweezers and scratching gently above the stinger, which removes the top layer of the skin so the stinger can be removed in its entirety. You can then apply Calamine or a paste of baking soda and water to decrease itching and to soothe the pain.

If part of the stinger is left in, it may precipitate an ongoing allergic response, so notify your doctor if that is the case.

Also notify your doctor if an insect bite or bee sting is associated with face or mouth swelling, problems breathing or wheezing, fever, or increasing swelling and redness despite the above treatment.

Choose an insect repellant with up to 30 percent DEET, and dress your child in protective clothing if you're in an area where there are a lot of mosquitoes or other insects. If she gets an insect bite that is very red, swollen, and itchy, you can give her oral Benadryl and place 1 percent cortisone cream. If she's stung by a bee, scratch out the stinger and apply Calamine or baking soda and water. Severe reactions to insect bites or bee stings are rare; however, call your doctor if your baby has face or mouth swelling, problems breathing, fever, or increased swelling and redness.

Last One in the Pool—Fun in the Water

One of the most enjoyable yet dangerous activities during the summer is swimming—or, if you're a baby, just having fun in the water. Parents often ask me: "When can we take our baby in a swimming pool, in the ocean, or in the lake? Is chlorine dangerous? Is it true babies naturally hold their breath underwater?" Here is my advice on how to make sure you and your young child enjoy the water safely.

Infants can go in the water at any age. It doesn't matter whether it is the ocean, a lake, a river, or a swimming pool. Chlorine and other chemicals in the pool will not hurt your baby nor will saltwater; however, there are several other factors to consider:

1. *Water temperature:* Infants have less subcutaneous fat and thus less protection from changes in temperature than we do. So if the water is cold, your baby will get cold quicker than you will. You'll need to monitor how cold she's getting. If she feels cold or is shivering, or if she gets fussy, take her out of the water and warm her up.

2. *Sun exposure:* The sun reflects off the water, giving your baby more intense exposure to the sun, even if you are just wading in the water. Make sure she is wearing adequate sunscreen as well as a T-shirt and hat.

3. *Dry skin:* Water dries out the skin so it's not a bad idea to moisturize your baby's skin when you get out of the water.

4. *Drowning:* Obviously, this is the most serious concern. It's true that infants are born with a breath-holding reflex, which allows them to hold their breath when their head is submerged underwater. However, this is not a party trick that you should try on your own. Your child may go under the water and come up fine, but she may also take a breath at the wrong time, gasp, choke, and flood her lungs. Despite the breath-holding reflex, no child truly understands water safety, nor does the reflex protect her against accidental drowning. You should never dunk your infant under the water unless supervised by a professional. *As for water wings:* they're fun but not true lifesaving devices. A baby's arms stay afloat, but not the head. So even when she's wearing them, your child still needs to be closely supervised.

Common Sense Bottom Line
Enjoying the water is fine whether it's in the ocean, lakes, streams, or pools. Just don't forget sun protection, remember to take her out of the water and warm her up if she's getting too cold, and no dunking!

Fun with Cats and Dogs—Exposing Your Baby to Pets

When I married my wife I got more than a loving bride; I got her cat, our first baby. When my wife was about eight months pregnant we noticed that the cat was growing very clingy. He would follow us around the house constantly, meow, rub up against our legs, and sleep on our bed, all of which he had never done before. He knew something was up: a demotion was looming. Many new parents with pets have had a similar experience before or shortly after returning home with their new baby. And new moms and dads often ask, *Do I need to keep my child away from my dog or cat to avoid a possible allergic reaction?*

The answer may surprise you. Early exposure to dogs and cats may actually *decrease* your child's risk of allergy to pets later on in life, so it may be beneficial to have your child roll around with

Fluffy. With that said, even if your dog is as mellow as Lassie, all pets are unpredictable. Dogs and cats can get easily excited or scared and may nip, bite, or scratch your baby by accident. Unfortunately, this could lead to a serious injury in an infant. Rather than worrying about itchy eyes and sneezing, cuddle up with your baby next to Fido or Fluffy, but supervise the visit.

Common Sense Bottom Line
Don't worry about your baby's exposure to your pet; it's a good thing. It will decrease her risk of later allergic reactions. Do supervise her playtime with your cat or dog to prevent accidental bites or scratches.

Are We There Yet?—Traveling with Your Baby

Technically, your child is safe to travel anytime after she has been discharged from the hospital after delivery. While most families like to settle in for a while before taking off on vacation, when you do decide to travel with your baby, it's good to have a sense of what's okay and what's not.

Should you decide to travel on a plane, there's no need to worry about potential problems with her ears adjusting to the altitude. Taking her on a plane is perfectly safe. However, I recommend waiting to fly, if possible, until after she has had her first set of vaccinations, because airports and airplanes are environments where she's likely to be exposed to infections. If you do take your baby on a plane trip, here are some safety tips:

1. Carry the baby in a covered car seat or hold her so that she's facing your body and breathing on you. This will keep her away from people who are coughing and sneezing.
2. Try to get a window seat and place her there. Even though the air on a plane is recycled, at least she'll be positioned farthest from other passengers in the cabin.
3. Try to time her breast or bottle feedings so they coincide with take-offs and landings. Swallowing helps to clear her ears.

(Pacifiers don't work as well because the baby doesn't swallow as much.)

4. If she's sleeping, don't wake her up to feed her during the take-off or landing—or for any reason. Sleeping peacefully is a good thing.

5. Make the trip fun by bringing along a few distracting toys. Most babies have no clue that they are on a plane and don't feel any different en route. So relax . . . and enjoy the ride!

More flight tips for traveling with your baby:

1. Once your baby can crawl or walk, I suggest that, if you can afford it, you reserve a separate seat for your child, especially for longer trips. This will allow her space to fall asleep comfortably in her car seat rather than attempting to fall asleep on Mom or Dad.

2. Don't forget to bring the car seat.

3. Tell the airline that you are flying with an infant, and it will try to reserve seats in the bulkhead section. A bulkhead is nice, because you'll have extra room to put your baby on the floor to crawl and play.

Daddy vs. Doctor—Flying High on the Red Eye

Before we had our own child, my wife and I would joke that if there was a screaming child anywhere in the airport waiting area, the little darling was destined to be seated within one row of us. Call it the luck of the pediatrician. On the plane, I remember watching families with crying children and feeling bad for them because I knew there was nothing they could do. If a baby doesn't want to be cooped up for hours on an airplane, she's going to let you know. I would also notice the looks other people would shoot the exasperated parents: empathetic or hostile, probably depending on who had children and who didn't.

Then it came time for us to take our first flight with

Aubrey, who was then five months old. It seemed like a great age to fly, because Aubrey wasn't mobile yet, so she would sit on our laps happily. Also, my wife was breastfeeding, so we had the ultimate soothing measure at our disposal whenever it was needed. Still, we were worried. Were we going to become *those* people who annoy an entire planeful of passengers with a fussy baby? How much stuff could we bring and not hold up the security line? How could we coordinate carrying the baby, the car seat, the stroller, a diaper bag, and toys to keep her busy?

At the airport, we checked in early, made it through security in record time, and even received compliments on how organized we were as a family. We were a well-oiled machine. Then we got to the gate and the looks started. I could tell everyone was thinking the same thing: *This is a red eye—please don't let that baby sit anywhere near me.*

Once on the plane, we had our plan all worked out. Try to feed Aubrey during take-off, and she'd easily fall asleep— and hopefully sleep most of the way there. It didn't quite work out that way. She started to get fussy as we taxied to the runway, so my wife put her on the breast early. She did fall asleep, but we were still on the ground. Then we sat on the runway for twenty minutes while the pilot kept making announcements to update us. Those announcements were so loud that each time his voice barreled through the speaker, Aubrey woke up. Upon take-off: another announcement. Upon reaching cruising altitude: another announcement. When beverage service was about to begin: yet another. And the same with the headsets announcement and the movie preview announcement.

All I can say is: thank goodness for breastfeeding. Aubrey finally got to sleep despite all the noisy interruptions. And there were no hostile looks from any of our fellow travelers.

I can't say the same for her second flight, when Aubrey

was nine months old. No nine-month-old will sit in your lap for six hours, and Aubrey was no different. She wanted to be walked up and down the aisle constantly to check out what was going on. My wife and I took turns trying to find people who looked like sympathetic grandparents and didn't mind making funny faces at Aubrey to make her smile during these strolls.

When it was time for her to go to sleep, she didn't cry, but she couldn't get comfortable because my wife and I had to keep passing her back and forth as she tried to lie across our laps. Breastfeeding wasn't working this time either, as my wife tried it at least ten times in an hour with no success. There were no outright mean looks from the other passengers, but there was definitely some uncomfortable baby whining going on, which wasn't really Aubrey's fault. We learned a few lessons on that trip, though.

Baby Boob Tube?—Should Your Baby Watch TV?

Current American Academy of Pediatrics guidelines recommend that children do not watch television for the first two years of life, advocating instead parental involvement in the form of talking, singing, reading, listening to music, or playing. Why is that? Do I believe that TV causes ADHD? No. But we do know that 3-D learning is always better than 2-D learning.

When your child sits in front of the television, she does the same thing you do: veg out. You may think she's enthralled by the Baby Einstein program you've switched on for her to watch while you get some housework done. But the fact is she's not learning anything; she is just watching images move by like a big screen saver. Videos such as Baby Einstein have been shown to inhibit a child's verbal IQ because every hour your baby spends in front of the television is an hour she is not receiving verbal stimulation from you. The more words that are spoken to your child by an actual person, the more words she hears "live and in person," the better her speech and language development will be.

That being said, I don't think there's any harm if your child sits on your lap while you watch a ball game or your favorite episode of *Scrubs*. Just make sure to talk to her while you're watching your show. Every morning my wife and I enjoy sitting with Aubrey and watching *Sesame Street*, a ritual I remember enjoying with my parents as a child. And Aubrey has definitely learned from watching the show. The key is to interact with her as you would when you read her a book. Ask her questions, tell her what you're seeing on the tube, and be as involved with her as you are in the program. The point is to refrain from using the TV as a babysitter.

Common Sense Bottom Line
Babies just want to have fun—and your baby has more fun with you than with the boob tube.

Time for Number Two—Tips for Introducing the Second Child

Now that you are cruising through the first year, you might think, *Let's do it all again.* With the excitement of a new child will come new questions. How are you going to breastfeed your newborn with your first climbing on top of you? How are you going to be able to watch both of them at the same time? How do you carry all of the "baby stuff"? What if the baby cries and wakes up the older child? She was just becoming a good sleeper. And what is she going to think of the new baby? Here are some ways to make the transition to number two, three, or four easier on number one.

Before Arrival
- *Reinforce the idea that a baby is coming.* Having a baby is an abstract idea to an infant or toddler, so the topic needs to be revisited over and over again. When your baby bump begins to be noticeable to others, start using phrases such

as "there's a baby in Mommy's belly" or "you are going to be a great big sister."

- *A picture is worth a thousand words.* Show her pictures of when she was a baby and talk to her about how she is a big girl now.

- *Let her feel your stomach.* All the while, reinforcing the ideas of being a big sister and how lucky the baby is going to be to have a big sister like her.

- *Get her involved.* Let her be involved in the preparation for the new baby (if she seems interested). Allow her to help decorate the new baby's room. Pull out old toys and stuffed animals that she would like to share with the new baby. Don't be surprised if she becomes territorial with the same things that she was not interested in just a few months before.

In the Hospital

- *She misses you the most.* If she is going to visit you (and the new baby) in the hospital, place your newborn in the nursery. Even the most excited older sibling still misses you, and if she walks in and sees you holding a new baby then, the new baby has already replaced her in her mind. If you have Dad or the nurse bring the baby into the room, then the new baby will be perceived as a gift for the whole family.

- *Reinforce the idea that she is a wonderful big sister.* As soon as the new baby enters the room, start using phrases such as "you are such a good big sister," "you are so gentle," and "your brother is lucky to have such a great big sister." Don't be surprised when she tests boundaries to see how she can get your attention. The most common behavior is hitting her new baby brother or sister. She does not really want to hurt the baby, she just wants to see at what point you will pay attention to her. For example, she will sit down next to the new baby and pat her gently, then she will turn and look directly at you and the patting will become harder and harder until it is a hit or slap. By giving her tons of attention from the get-go she will not need to escalate her behavior to get your attention in a negative way.

- *Place familiar objects in the room.* Place a couple pictures of her on the side of the new baby's bassinet. This will reinforce the idea that she is important. Also, give her a present "from the new baby" and have her choose one she can give to her sibling. This act reinforces sharing and may distract an already overwhelmed big sister.

- *Give more attention.* Make sure everyone who visits you, whether it be at the hospital or at home, walks right over to her, bends down and says hello before they give attention to the new baby. The new baby will not know nor care if he is ignored, but trust me, she will. Imagine that everyone used to walk in the room and dote over you, and now they just walk right past you to someone else. What a horrible feeling.

At Home

- *Keep your one-on-one time.* If Mom always reads a story to her, then keep doing that. If Dad always takes her to the park, then keep doing that. Keep as much of your old routine as possible so she is still receiving as much of your one-on-one attention and so everything does not revolve around the four of you. It may actually feel as if she is receiving more attention then ever before and the new baby is being neglected. Of course, you should do activities as a family as well, but it is important to make her feel as important as possible. I have seen older siblings appear to be very excited about the new baby, then ask their parents a couple days later "Baby go home now?" When the parents replied, "Baby is home now," their daughter retorted, "No, baby go to another home now," as if the baby were a new doll she was done playing with.

- *Everyone loves presents.* Keep little gifts at home for her. Every visitor is going to bring a gift for the new baby and many will forget to bring something for the older sibling.

- *Give her jobs and make her feel responsible.* Remember,

everything you do with the new baby (feed him, change his diaper, pick him up when he is crying) is attention taken away from her. That is why many older siblings regress to wanting their bottle again, wearing diapers, or sleeping in a crib—they feel this is a good way to get your attention. When you are breastfeeding do not be surprised if she wants to climb on top of you, so give her a job. Tell her, "You know what would really help Mommy, if you put your hand on my knee," or "Honey, can you get me a diaper for your baby brother." There may be times, however, that you just have to say "Mommy is busy right now and she will play with you after," no matter how mad she gets.

- *Even the playing field.* My all-time favorite way to tip the balance for attention is to reprimand the new baby in front of her. For example, if you are playing with her and the baby cries, say out loud, "I am playing with your sister right now, I will be with you in a second." You will actually see her puff up and smile as if to say, "Yeah, I am more important."

Remember, this is a new transition for everyone, and over time everything will fall into place. Now that you have the knowledge of number one under your belt, number two will be a breeze.

Daddy vs. Doctor—Number Two

The night before my wife, Aubrey, and I were leaving for vacation, I walked into the bathroom and saw two pregnancy tests sitting on the counter. Each strip had parallel pink lines. I looked at my wife, surprised, and said, "You're pregnant! Oh, man, this means you can't drink on vacation?" My wife's smile dissolved. I could have said a million more appropriate things but didn't. *I am so excited. Aubrey is going to make a great big sister. This is perfect. I love you.* Instead, I had to stick my foot in my mouth. My wife looked at me and said sarcastically, "I'm glad you're so excited." I was excited, but a wave of anxiety overcame me. We had been trying for only a short time. Aubrey was only fourteen months old and she was my girl. I did not feel like I had had enough one-on-one time with her. We had a daily routine and she slept through the night. She was my little sidekick and everything was perfect. I guess I was just scared of anything that could disrupt that. I realized that being a doctor and a daddy did not mean that I was immune to feeling scared or anxious when it came to being a new parent. I now understood that another baby would mean a whole new set of experiences, but Aubrey would still be my little girl—and I will have a new love that I could not imagine life without.

AFTERWORD

. . . .

I've heard parenting described thusly: "The days are long but the years are short." Long days because when you have a new baby all the days run into each other. Short years because before you know it your child will be graduating high school and leaving for college. Time passes quickly, and it is important to take advantage of every moment and enjoy yourself.

With the responsibility, emotions, and demands that come with having a baby, life can seem complicated, and it may be easy to get overwhelmed. All you want is what is best for her. Unfortunately, the yearning to do everything perfectly often results in anxiety and stress about *not* doing it perfectly. Keep life with your baby simple. Trust your instincts and use common sense as your guide. Imagine there was no Internet. Imagine there was nobody to call in the middle of the night for advice. Imagine you lost your cable connection. Now imagine you are alone at night and your child starts to cry inconsolably. What would you do? Your natural parenting instincts would take over and you and your child would be okay. And after reading this book you have the added knowledge to handle these situations with confidence.

So the next time someone gives you advice or tells you the tenth different way to do something just smile and say "thank you." Go home, process the information, and do what works best for you and your family. Decide for yourself. There is not always one right way to do something. Your child trusts you, now you just need to trust yourself. Laugh at watery poop. Smile at projectile spit-up. Blame your husband for the baby's bad gas and bring the fun back into raising your child.

ACKNOWLEDGMENTS

. . . .

When I began writing this book, I remember thinking to myself, *How hard can it be? I give this advice every day. All I need to do is write it down on paper.* Boy, was I wrong. I have gained an immense respect for all writers and their craft. This book could not have been completed without the support and guidance of many important people; like raising a child, it truly does take a village.

Eat, Sleep, Poop has been molded by people throughout my life. My parents have shaped how I see myself as a father and empowered me to pursue a career in medicine. Without their unwavering support and love, this book would not have been possible.

My own pediatrician, Dr. Frank Stroud, had to tell me at the age of twenty-one that I needed to graduate to an adult doctor after watching me try to squeeze onto a small waiting room chair (made for a five-year-old). His bedside manner and healing touch inspired me to become a pediatrician.

Without Chris Fenton I never would have gotten this book off the ground. He introduced me to my literary agency, Venture Literary, and my wonderful literary agent, Jennifer de la Fuente. Jennifer has gone above and beyond her duties as an agent in supporting this book. She guided me throughout the process and helped to shape and reshape the book as it evolved from a book proposal to the final text. She read every line of every draft and stood behind my vision from the beginning. She was also responsible for connecting me with Samantha Martin at Scribner. Sam worked tirelessly and has patiently put up with all of my questions as a first-time author. The support I received from Scribner has made writing *Eat, Sleep, Poop* an enjoyable experience and I appreciate all of their hard work and insight.

Eat, Sleep, Poop would also not have been complete without the invaluable editing and feedback of a host of friends, family, and colleagues. Dr. William La Via added both his medical expertise as a pediatric infectious disease specialist and his own personal experience as a father of two. My good friend and old college roommate from Cornell University, Daniel Dornbusch, added his "I don't have a kid yet but someday will" point of view. Haley Fisher, a talented writer and mother of two, contributed her "I have been there done that" perspective as both a mother and a writer. Alan Sitomer, father and author, added advice and feedback on the writing process. Laura Bellotti contributed her expertise as both an editor and a mother. John Baudino, father-to-be, lent his computer expertise to make sure the flow diagrams were both visually appealing and accurate. Dr. Bess Raker, pediatrician and co-founder of Beverly Hills Pediatrics, and Dr. Karen Hovav, pediatrician, graciously volunteered to read chapters and provided feedback. My colleagues at both Cedars-Sinai Medical Center and Children's Hospital Los Angeles have been a source of inspiration and support during my career. I would like to give special thanks to Dr. Kenneth Wright, pediatric ophthalmologist, and Dr. Andrew Freedman, pediatric urologist, for their expertise in their respective fields. I also greatly appreciate the patients of Beverly Hills Pediatrics for supporting our practice and me. I have been so fortunate to be part of the lives of so many wonderful families.

My greatest thanks must go to two very special people—my daughter Aubrey and my wife, Erin, without whom I would not have been able to write this book. It was truly a journey of learning throughout our first year together as new parents. Aubrey helped to shape how I practice as a pediatrician and how I follow through with my advice as a father. She taught me how to be a better daddy and doctor and about the true meaning of common sense parenting. Finally, thank you to my wife and "coauthor," Erin, who is probably sick and tired of reading this book and hearing me ask, "Will you just listen to this one line and tell me if it sounds okay?" I know she can recite this book from cover to cover and has been more than patient with the time demand it placed on our family. She allowed me to poke fun at our experiences as new parents and share our successes and struggles. She is the perfect partner and mother.

NOTE ON SOURCES

. . . .

The practice of medicine is constantly evolving. As a physician, it is important not only to stay up to date with current practices but to also question old ones. As I wrote this book, I drew from a myriad of personal and professional experiences. I used lessons I learned while working at both Childrens Hospital Los Angeles and Cedars-Sinai Medical Center, while caring for children from birth to adolescence in the newborn nursery, pediatric ward, as well as the neonatal and pediatric intensive care units. I adopted views that were shaped by colleagues and teaching attendings that continue to influence me in my career. I have also drawn from my experiences interacting with patients and their families in private practice and from the practical experience of being a new dad.

As the world of pediatrics changes, so, too, have many of my own recommendations to patients. Some of these changes come solely from scientific proof while others are a blend of science and my own personal experiences. For example, I only recently started advising patients that it is okay to try peanut products before the age of one based on recent articles and consultation with pediatric allergy specialists suggesting that it is both safe and possibly beneficial. After watching my daughter Aubrey enjoy countless strawberries and tomatoes at nine months old I became more lax on the previous recommendations to wait until one year to introduce these foods because of concerns over allergies. Sure, she developed a facial rash of the sort I warn parents about, but it wasn't serious and it went away shortly after she finished eating. Most important, it didn't bother her so why should I let it bother me?

When I look for the most up-to-date pediatric advice, I search the current recommendations from trusted organizations such as the American Academy of Pediatrics (www.aap.org) and the Centers for Disease Control and Prevention (www.cdc.gov). For example, the American Academy of Pediatrics' policy statements on breast-feeding and the vitamin K injection are useful resources for further information. I also used prestigious pediatric medical journals such as *Pediatrics* and articles from *Infectious Diseases in Children* as the basis of information on such topics as umbilical cord care, cord blood banking, vaccines, and the universal newborn hearing screen.

For a controversial topic such as vaccines, it is especially important to research all sides of the story. It is not enough to just read scientific texts, I also want to understand where my patients are getting their information and what books they are reading. I think it is difficult to have a productive or intelligent conversation about a topic unless you understand the origin of both sides of the argument. As a result, I researched several different sources from celebrity books to scientific papers. I reviewed texts with points of view both for and against vaccines. I drew from current news articles including a March 2009 *Los Angeles Times* article discussing the rise in nonvaccinated children in California, a March 2009 *New York Times* article on the public health risk seen as parents reject vaccines, and a *Time* article on a genetic link to autism. I reviewed multiple scientific studies in medical journals written by infectious disease experts such as Dr. Paul Offit, the director of the Vaccine Education Center at Children's Hospital of Philadelphia, and personally discussed topics with other pediatric infectious disease specialists.

Common Sense Bottom Line

This book would not be complete without weeding through multiple sources, taking into account past experiences, heeding lessons learned from trusted advisers, and, of course, a little common sense.

REFERENCES

How to Use the References

For easy reference, in this section I'm including duplicates of the fact sheets and diagnosis and treatment diagrams I have used throughout the book. These reference sheets will help you easily decipher and appropriately treat your child's symptoms. Feel free to tear out or photocopy the following pages and carry them with you in your diaper bag, hang them on your refrigerator, or share them with a friend.

Newborn Must-Haves Checklist

Sleep
___ Crib
___ Crib mattress
___ Mattress pad cover
___ Fitted sheet

Travel
___ Car seat
___ Stroller
___ Diaper bag

Clothing
___ Onesies/sleepers
___ Swaddling blanket

Changing

___ Changing table with pad/soft rug or mat
___ Diapers
___ Gauze/baby wipes
___ Diaper cream

Bath/Hygiene

___ Infant bathing basin
___ Sponge/washcloth
___ Baby soap and moisturizer
___ Nail file/clippers

Medications

___ Infant and children's acetaminophen (Tylenol)
___ Children's diphenhydramine (Benadryl)
___ Electrolyte replacement fluid (Pedialyte)
___ Antigas/colic remedies (Mylicon, Gripe water, Hyland's Colic Tabs)
___ Sunscreen
___ Insect repellant

Accessories

___ Digital thermometer (rectal and axillary/underarm)
___ Pacifier
___ Bulb syringe
___ Saline nasal spray
___ Gum/tooth cleansers
___ Hand sanitizer

Feeding

___ Bottles (4 ounces)
___ Nipples (level one)
___ Breast pump
___ Freezer bags
___ Nursing pads
___ Nursing bra

Pediatrician Checklist

Name of Doctor/Office: _____

	Not important				Very Important
Office size					
___Small (three or fewer doctors)	1	2	3	4	5
___Large (more than three doctors)	1	2	3	4	5
Gender					
___Male	1	2	3	4	5
___Female	1	2	3	4	5
Age					
___Young	1	2	3	4	5
___Old	1	2	3	4	5
Board certification	1	2	3	4	5
Availability/office hours					
___Weekend hours	1	2	3	4	5
___Nighttime hours	1	2	3	4	5
Access to doctor					
___Via phone	1	2	3	4	5
___Via e-mail	1	2	3	4	5
___Office visits only	1	2	3	4	5
Who sees you in the office?					
___Your doctor	1	2	3	4	5
___Another doctor in the practice	1	2	3	4	5
___Physician assistant	1	2	3	4	5
___Nurse	1	2	3	4	5
Who takes after-hours calls?					
___Your practice	1	2	3	4	5
___Shares with another pediatric group	1	2	3	4	5

___Nursing triage or hospital	1	2	3	4	5
___No one	1	2	3	4	5
Overall philosophy					
___Western medicine	1	2	3	4	5
___Homeopathic/holistic	1	2	3	4	5
Personality	1	2	3	4	5
Ancillary services					
___In-house lab	1	2	3	4	5
___Informative website	1	2	3	4	5
___Access to specialists	1	2	3	4	5
Staff					
___Not friendly (1)/most friendly (5)	1	2	3	4	5
___Physician assistants	1	2	3	4	5
___Registered nurses (RN)	1	2	3	4	5
___Licensed vocational nurses (LVN)	1	2	3	4	5
___Medical assistants	1	2	3	4	5
Facilities	1	2	3	4	5
Financial responsibility					
___Takes your insurance (in network)	1	2	3	4	5
___Fee for service (out of network)	1	2	3	4	5
___Bills for you	1	2	3	4	5
Hospital Affiliation					
___Visits your newborn in the hospital after birth	1	2	3	4	5
Punctuality	1	2	3	4	5

Medications Safe for Use by Breastfeeding Mothers

Acyclovir

Advil (ibuprofen)

Albuterol

Allopurinol

Amoxicillin

Ampicillin

Ancef (cefazolin)

Atrovent

Augmenin

Bactrim/Septra (after two
    months old)

Bactroban (mupirocin)

Barium

Benadryl
    (diphenhydramine)

Biaxin (clarithromycin)

Ceftin (cefuroxime)

Cefzil (cefprozil)

Ciprofloxacin

Claritin (loratidine)

Colace (docusate)

Coumadin (warfarin)

Dextromethorphan

Diflucan (fluconazole)

Domperidone

Elimite (permethrin)

Erythromycin

Fluoride

Gentamicin

Heparin

Hydrocortisone Cream

Imitrex (sumatriptan)

Imodium (loperamide)

Insulin

Kaopectate

Keflex (cephalexin)

Maalox

Macrobid/Macrodantin
    (nitrofurantoin)

Milk of Magnesia

Monistat (miconazole)

Motrin (ibuprofen)

Nix (permethrin)

Nystatin

Omnicef (cefdinir)

Pepcid (famotidine)

Robitussin (guaifenesin)

Rocephin (ceftriaxone)

Scopolamine Patch

Suprax (cefixime)

Synthroid (levothyroxine)

Tagamet (cimetidine)

Tylenol (acetaminophen)

Valtrex (valacycolvir)

Xopenex (levalbuterol)

Zantac (ranitidine)

Zithromax (azithromycin)

Zyrtec (ceirizine)

Over-the-counter cough/
    cold/sore throat remedies

Miscellaneous

- Many herbal supplements have not been studied and as a result have not been approved by the FDA. Their effect on nursing babies is unknown.

- Many medications such as antidepressants (Prozac, Zoloft, Paxil) are in a category in which there are either no controlled studies in breastfeeding women or controlled studies show only minimal nonthreatening adverse effects. Because there are not enough studies to deem them "safe," each parent must weigh whether the potential benefit of taking the medication justifies the potential risk to the baby.

Milk Allergy Diagnosis and Treatment

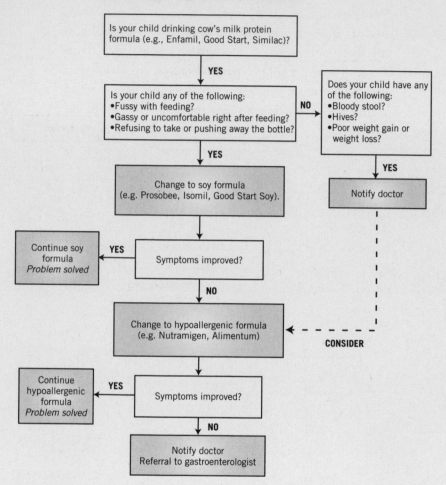

Crying at Random Times

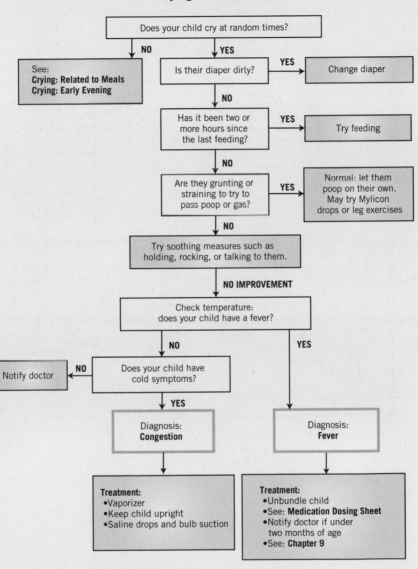

Does your child cry at random times?

NO →
See:
Crying: Related to Meals
Crying: Early Evening

YES ↓

Is their diaper dirty? — **YES** → Change diaper

NO ↓

Has it been two or more hours since the last feeding? — **YES** → Try feeding

NO ↓

Are they grunting or straining to try to pass poop or gas? — **YES** → Normal: let them poop on their own. May try Mylicon drops or leg exercises

NO ↓

Try soothing measures such as holding, rocking, or talking to them.

NO IMPROVEMENT ↓

Check temperature: does your child have a fever?

NO ↓   **YES** ↓

Does your child have cold symptoms? — **NO** → Notify doctor

YES ↓

Diagnosis: **Congestion**

Diagnosis: **Fever**

Treatment:
- Vaporizer
- Keep child upright
- Saline drops and bulb suction

Treatment:
- Unbundle child
- See: **Medication Dosing Sheet**
- Notify doctor if under two months of age
- See: **Chapter 9**

263

Crying Related to Meals

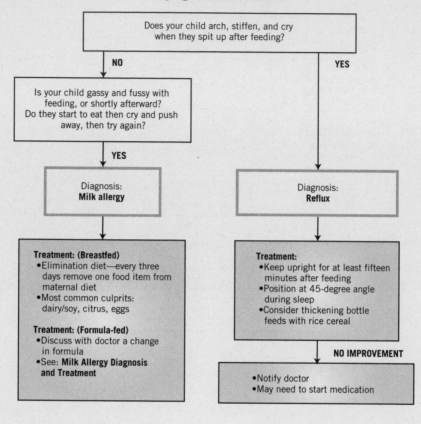

Does your child arch, stiffen, and cry
when they spit up after feeding?

NO

YES

Is your child gassy and fussy with
feeding, or shortly afterward?
Do they start to eat then cry and push
away, then try again?

YES

Diagnosis:
Milk allergy

Diagnosis:
Reflux

Treatment: (Breastfed)
• Elimination diet—every three
  days remove one food item from
  maternal diet
• Most common culprits:
  dairy/soy, citrus, eggs

Treatment: (Formula-fed)
• Discuss with doctor a change
  in formula
• See: **Milk Allergy Diagnosis
  and Treatment**

Treatment:
• Keep upright for at least fifteen
  minutes after feeding
• Position at 45-degree angle
  during sleep
• Consider thickening bottle
  feeds with rice cereal

NO IMPROVEMENT

• Notify doctor
• May need to start medication

264

Crying in the Early Evening (Two Weeks to Three Months of Age)

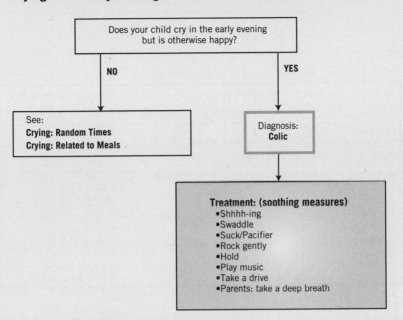

Does your child cry in the early evening but is otherwise happy?

NO

See:
Crying: Random Times
Crying: Related to Meals

YES

Diagnosis:
Colic

Treatment: (soothing measures)
- Shhhh-ing
- Swaddle
- Suck/Pacifier
- Rock gently
- Hold
- Play music
- Take a drive
- Parents: take a deep breath

Medication Dosing Sheet
Always use weight in determining dosage.
Use age only when weight is unknown.

Tylenol (to be given every four hours as needed)

Age	Weight	Infant drops (80mg/0.8ml)	Children's liquid susp (160mg/5ml)	Chewable tabs (80mg)
0–3 mos	6–11 lbs	0.4 ml	$1/4$ tsp	—
4–9 mos	12–15 lbs	0.8 ml	$1/2$ tsp	1 tab
9–12 mos	16–21 lbs	1.2 ml	$3/4$ tsp	1.5 tabs
12–23 mos	22–32 lbs	1.6 ml	1 tsp	2 tabs
2–3 yrs	33–40 lbs		$1 1/2$ tsps	3 tabs
4–5 yrs	41–54 lbs		2 tsps	4 tabs
6–8 yrs	55–64 lbs		$2 1/2$ tsps	5 tabs
9–10 yrs	65–88 lbs		3 tsps	6 tabs

Motrin (to be given every six hours as needed)

Do not give to children under six months.

Age	Weight	Infant drops (50mg/1.25ml)	Children's liquid susp (100mg/5ml)	Chew tabs (50mg)	Junior chewable tab (100mg)
6–9 mos	12–15 lbs	1.25 ml	$1/2$ tsp	1 tab	
9–12 mos	16–21 lbs	1.875 ml	$3/4$ tsp	$1 1/2$ tabs	
12–23 mos	22–32 lbs	2.5 ml	1 tsp	2 tabs	1 tab
2–3 yrs	33–40 lbs		$1 1/2$ tsps	3 tabs	$1 1/2$ tabs
4–5 yrs	41–54 lbs		2 tsps	4 tabs	2 tabs
6–8 yrs	55–64 lbs		$2 1/2$ tsps	5 tabs	$2 1/2$ tabs
9–10 yrs	65–88 lbs		3 tsps	6 tabs	3 tabs

Children's liquid preparations (cough, cold, and allergy medications such as Benadryl, Dimetapp, Triaminic, etc.)

Cough and cold medications are not *recommended under the age of four.*

Benadryl may be used in children under the age of four for allergy purposes only.

Age	Weight	Dose	Frequency
6–11 mos	12–17 lbs	$1/2$ tsp	every 6 hrs
1–2 yrs	18–30 lbs	1 tsp	every 6 hrs
3–6 yrs	31–44 lbs	$1^{1}/_{2}$ tsps	every 6 hrs
6–12 yrs	45 lbs and up	2 tsps	every 6 hrs

Common Sense Facts: Diarrhea

What is diarrhea? Diarrhea is defined as a sudden increase in watery stool. It is usually caused by a virus and may last one to two weeks. Diarrhea may present alone or with a combination of symptoms that include vomiting, fever, and fussiness. The symptoms are usually most severe in the first twenty-four to forty-eight hours.

Breastfed infants
- Provide breast milk on demand, which may be more frequently than normal.

Formula-fed infants
- Avoid cow's milk–based formulas that have lactose (Enfamil Lipil, Simalac Advance, Good Start Supreme) until normal stools resume.
- Soy-based (Prosobee, Isomil, Good Start Soy) or lactose-free formulas are okay.
- Offer oral rehydration solutions (Pedialyte) or other clear fluids. Water is okay if there is no vomiting.

If she is at the stage where she is eating solids
- Don't worry if she doesn't want to eat for several days. She'll lose weight but regain it when her appetite returns.
- Avoid dairy foods and fruit juices, as they may exacerbate the loose stools.
- Offer a well-balanced diet, but know it's okay if your child doesn't want to eat anything at all.
- Most important: lots of fluids will prevent a trip to the emergency room!

Call your doctor if
- Your baby doesn't urinate at least three times in twenty-four hours.
- There is blood in her stool.
- Your baby is inconsolable or has a fever for more than seventy-two hours.

Common Sense Facts: Fever

What Is Fever?

- Fever is your body's normal reaction to an infection—it is a good thing.
- Fever is a temperature of 100.4 degrees Fahrenheit or higher.
- A temperature of less than 100.4 is normal and does not need to be treated.

What Is the Best Way to Take a Baby's Temperature?

- Rectal temperatures are the most accurate and should always be used in babies under two months of age.
- An underarm temperature in children older than two months may be used.
- Ear thermometers are notoriously inaccurate and should not be used.

Should I Be Afraid of a Fever?

- *No!*
- Fever, whether it is 101 or 105, will not cause brain damage and will not hurt your child.
- How your child looks, acts, and feels when she does not have fever is more important than the number on the thermometer or how she looks when she has a fever.

Will Treating My Child's Fever Make the Infection Go Away?

- No, but it will make her feel better in the interim.

What Medicines Can I Use to Treat a Fever?

- Children younger than six months of age can be given Tylenol (acetaminophen) every four hours as needed.
- Children over six months of age can be given Tylenol every four hours or Motrin (ibuprofen) every six hours as needed.
- Tylenol and Motrin are two different medicines. Therefore, one medicine can be given between doses of the other medicine—if, and only if, the child's fever doesn't go down before her next dose of the first medicine.

269

- Tylenol and Motrin take approximately thirty minutes to an hour to work. Give the medicine time to work. See page 266 for a dosing chart.

Call Your Doctor If
- your baby is younger than two months of age and has a fever of 100.4 or higher.
- your child (of any age) has a fever that persists longer than seventy-two hours.
- your child's fever does not respond to Tylenol or Motrin.

Common Sense Facts: Colds
Symptoms of a Cold
- Coughing
- Sneezing
- Runny nose
- Nasal congestion
- Fever

Treatment
- Vaporizer or humidifier
- Steam shower
- Bulb suction and saline drops (sparingly)
- Lots of fluids
- Tylenol or Motrin for fever

What Not to Give Your Child
- Children under four years old should not be given over-the-counter cough/cold medicines.

Call Your Doctor If
- your baby's fever persists longer than seventy-two hours or it doesn't respond to the appropriate dose of Tylenol or Motrin.
- your baby has labored breathing.
- your baby has fewer than three wet diapers in a twenty-four-hour period.

Common Sense Facts: Croup

What Is Croup?

- Croup is a viral illness that causes fever and inflammation of the upper airway.
- When a child has croup, the airway below the vocal cords becomes swollen and narrow. This makes breathing noisy and difficult and causes a tight, barking cough. The cough is usually worse at night.

Who Gets It and How Long Does It Last?

- Children are most likely to get croup between six months and six years of age. After age six, it is not as common because the windpipe is larger, so swelling doesn't cause a problem.
- Some children get croup often.
- Croup can occur at any time of the year, but it is most common in the winter.
- Like any viral respiratory infection it can last for a week, but usually there are two bad nights of barking cough, and three days or fewer of fever.

What Can I Do to Help My Child?

- *Stay calm!* If you stay calm, your child will stay calm and breathe more comfortably.
- Sit with your baby in a steamy bathroom for five to ten minutes. Then take her out into the cold night air if available.
- Turn on a cool humidifier next to her crib.
- Use Tylenol or Motrin to bring down her fever.

Doesn't She Need Antibiotics or Medicine?

- As with other viruses, antibiotics are not an appropriate medicine.
- If your child continues to have labored raspy breathing she may need an oral steroid that your doctor will prescribe.

271

Should I Take Her to the Doctor or Emergency Room?
- Take her to the emergency room if she is having difficulty breathing even after trying the steamy shower and the cold-air walk/drive.
- If there is a history of breathing problems or prolonged fevers, see your doctor.

Common Sense Facts: Vomiting

Vomiting is usually caused by a viral infection and may last one to two weeks. Vomiting may be present alone or with a combination of symptoms that include diarrhea, fever, and fussiness. Treatment should be focused on supportive care and adequate hydration.

Breastfed infants
- Do not offer any solids or liquids for at least thirty to sixty minutes after vomiting.
- Provide breast milk in smaller amounts (shorter feedings) and more frequently than usual.

Formula-fed infants
- Do not offer any solids or liquids for at least thirty to sixty minutes after vomiting.
- Offer oral rehydration solutions (Pedialyte) or other clear liquids such as sugar water or tea.
- Offer small amounts frequently, gradually increasing the volume. For example, 1 teaspoon, then a couple minutes later another teaspoon, then a couple minutes later 2 teaspoons, and so on.
- If your child vomits while you are increasing the volume, wait another thirty to sixty minutes and start again.
- After four hours of no vomiting, you may return to formula.
- Avoid plain water. (Your body needs electrolytes; water may cause more vomiting.)

If she is at the stage where she is eating solids
- Do not worry if she does not want to eat anything.
- She may lose weight—this is normal, and she will gain it back when she is feeling better.
- Adequate hydration is the most important issue.

Common mistakes in the treatment of vomiting
- Giving liquids or solids too soon (especially water).
- Allowing your child to drink as much as she wants after vomiting instead of starting with small amounts and gradually increasing the volume.
- Using over-the-counter medication.

Call your doctor if
- your baby does not urinate at least three times in a twenty-four-hour period.
- there is blood in the vomit.
- your baby has a fever for more than seventy-two hours.
- your baby is inconsolable.

Rash Localized to Diaper Area
Diagnosis and Treatment

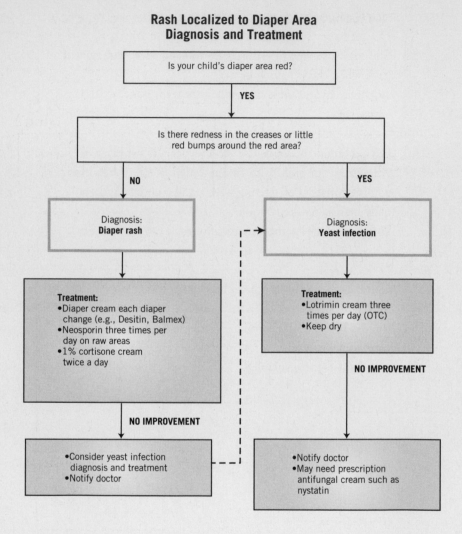

Is your child's diaper area red?

YES

Is there redness in the creases or little red bumps around the red area?

NO

Diagnosis:
Diaper rash

Treatment:
- Diaper cream each diaper change (e.g., Desitin, Balmex)
- Neosporin three times per day on raw areas
- 1% cortisone cream twice a day

NO IMPROVEMENT

- Consider yeast infection diagnosis and treatment
- Notify doctor

YES

Diagnosis:
Yeast infection

Treatment:
- Lotrimin cream three times per day (OTC)
- Keep dry

NO IMPROVEMENT

- Notify doctor
- May need prescription antifungal cream such as nystatin

Rash Localized to Creases/Skin Folds Diagnosis and Treatment

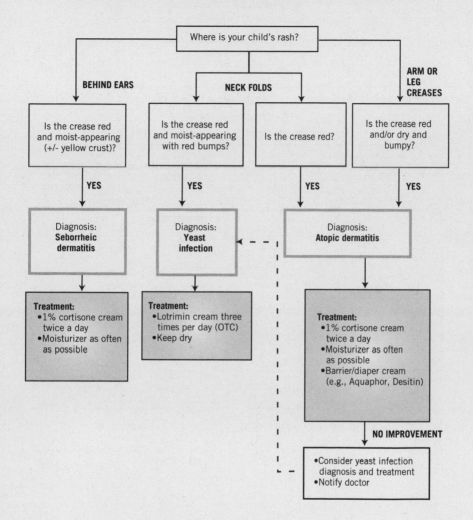

Rash Localized to Scalp Diagnosis and Treatment

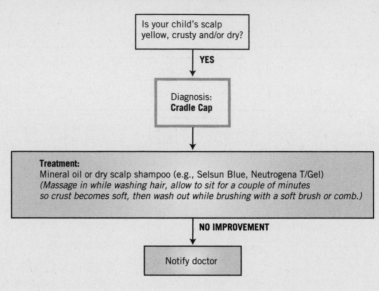

Is your child's scalp
yellow, crusty and/or dry?

YES

Diagnosis:
Cradle Cap

Treatment:
Mineral oil or dry scalp shampoo (e.g., Selsun Blue, Neutrogena T/Gel)
*(Massage in while washing hair, allow to sit for a couple of minutes
so crust becomes soft, then wash out while brushing with a soft brush or comb.)*

NO IMPROVEMENT

Notify doctor

Generalized Rash Diagnosis and Treatment

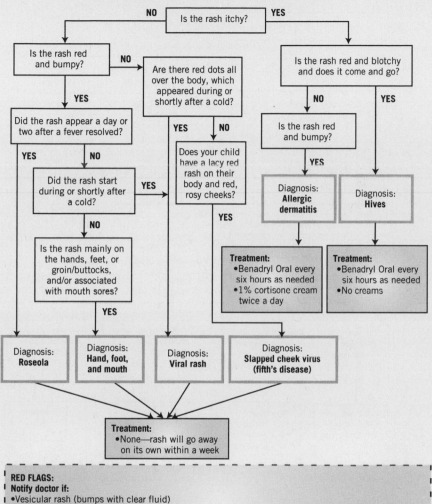

RED FLAGS:
Notify doctor if:
• Vesicular rash (bumps with clear fluid)
• Nonblanching rash—if you press on the red dots and they do not disappear (as if you dotted her with a red felt-tip pen)
• Child appears very sick (you think she needs to go to the emergency department or see the doctor immediately)

Ear Complaint Diagnosis and Treatment

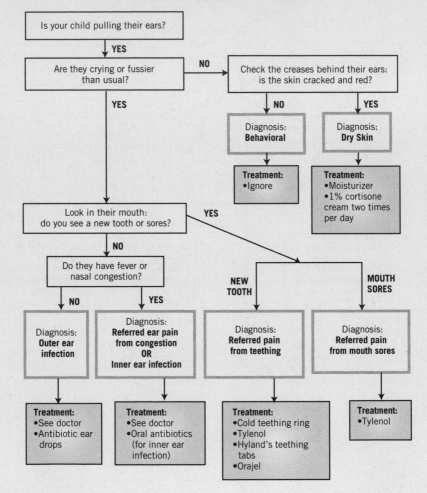

Is your child pulling their ears?

↓ **YES**

Are they crying or fussier than usual? → **NO** → Check the creases behind their ears: is the skin cracked and red?

↓ **YES** (from "crying or fussier")

NO → Diagnosis: **Behavioral** → Treatment: •Ignore

YES → Diagnosis: **Dry Skin** → Treatment: •Moisturizer •1% cortisone cream two times per day

Look in their mouth: do you see a new tooth or sores?

YES → NEW TOOTH / MOUTH SORES

↓ **NO**

Do they have fever or nasal congestion?

NO → Diagnosis: **Outer ear infection** → Treatment: •See doctor •Antibiotic ear drops

YES → Diagnosis: **Referred ear pain from congestion OR Inner ear infection** → Treatment: •See doctor •Oral antibiotics (for inner ear infection)

NEW TOOTH → Diagnosis: **Referred pain from teething** → Treatment: •Cold teething ring •Tylenol •Hyland's teething tabs •Orajel

MOUTH SORES → Diagnosis: **Referred pain from mouth sores** → Treatment: •Tylenol

278

Eye Complaint Diagnosis and Treatment

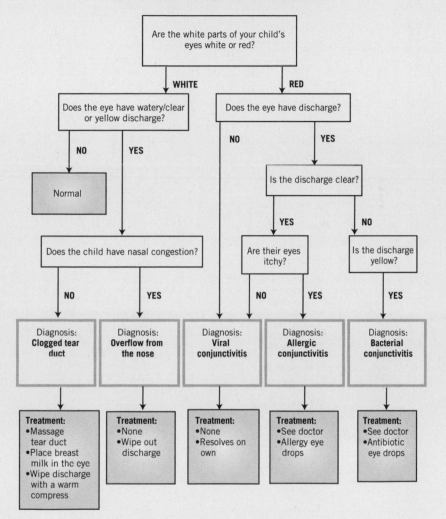

INDEX

ABOUT THE AUTHOR

· ·

Scott W. Cohen, M.D., F.A.A.P., is a board-certified pediatrician and the cofounder of Beverly Hills Pediatrics, where he currently practices. He is also an attending and active member of the teaching staff of Cedars Sinai Medical Center, where he was awarded Pediatrician of the Year in 2006 and was the recipient of the Physician Recognition Award in Pediatrics in 2005 and 2008. He completed his pediatric training in 2003 at the Childrens Hospital Los Angeles. There, he was the recipient of the Victor E. Stork Award for continued excellence and future promise in the care of children and the Associates and Affiliates award for scientific knowledge, clinical judgment, and excellence in human relations. He was also selected as one of the Best Doctors in America® 2007–2008 and 2009–2010. He lives in Los Angeles with his wife and daughter.